Laugh Aerobics

A practical guide to creating
your own laughter and humour

HELENE GROVER

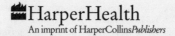

HarperHealth
An imprint of HarperCollins*Publishers*

This book is dedicated to my big brother Phillip, who was such a vital part of my childhood.

HarperHealth
An imprint of HarperCollins*Publishers*, Australia

First published in Australia in 1996
by HarperCollins*Publishers* Pty Limited
ACN 009 913 517
A member of the HarperCollins*Publishers* (Australia) Pty Limited Group

HarperCollins*Publishers*
25 Ryde Road, Pymble, Sydney NSW 2073, Australia
31 View Road, Glenfield, Auckland 10, New Zealand
77–85 Fulham Palace Road, London W6 8JB, United Kingdom
Hazelton Lanes, 55 Avenue Road, Suite 2900, Toronto, Ontario, M5R 3L2
and 1995 Markham Road, Scarborough, Ontario M1B 5M8, Canada
10 East 53rd Street, New York NY 10032, USA

The National Library of Australia Cataloguing-in-Publication data:

Grover, Helene.
   Laugh aerobics : a practical guide to creating your own
   laughter and humour.

   ISBN 0 7322 5615 1.

   1. Laughter – Therapeutic use. 2. Laughter – Psychological aspects. I. Title.

   152.4

Designed by Rosemarie Franzoni
Cover design by Rosemarie Franzoni
Cover and text illustrations by Neryl Walker
Typeset in Australia by Kimberly Williams
Printed in Australia by Griffin Paperbacks

9 8 7 6 5 4 3 2 1
99 98 97 96

Our thanks go to those who have given us permission to reproduce copyright material in this book. Particular sources of print material are acknowledged in the text. Every effort has been made to contact the copyright holders of print material, and the publisher welcomes communication from any copyright holder from whom permission was inadvertently not gained.

About the author

Since 1990, Australia's best-known laughter therapist, Helene Grover, has been running highly effective workshops and courses aimed at helping people bring more laughter and fun into their lives, thereby improving their mental and physical health.

In a sense, Helene has been preparing since childhood for this work. The personal difficulties she experienced in her early years have led her to cultivate a positive philosophy about life and to find humour and joy in almost every situation.

Born in Paris in 1942, Helene was the daughter of a Polish mother raised in Germany, and a Russian father. Both her parents were active in the French underground. The family stayed on in France after the war; they emigrated to Australia when Helene was nine, leaving behind her older brother.

A year after their arrival in Sydney, her father died of cancer. Helene's mother, illiterate and alone in a strange country, went out to work. In addition to going to school, Helene acted for many years as her caretaker, business manager, translator and companion.

In her early twenties, Helene surprised everyone – including herself – by writing a song that became a big hit: 'Barefoot Boy'. Its words encapsulated something of what she would later go on to celebrate in her work – the value of laughter and a deep appreciation of nature.

Over the following years Helene married, divorced, travelled overseas and worked at many office jobs. In her late twenties, she began an acting career and went on to found the highly successful Sydney Youth Workshop, a young people's creative drama group whose productions incorporated comedy and humour.

Eventually Helene opened her own theatrical agency. When one of 'her' comics told her that having her in his audience 'got everyone going', she realised how much she enjoyed laughing – heartily and noisily – and that she could favourably affect others.

Helene's sense of humour was mislaid in the course of a long-lasting and traumatic personal relationship that diminished her self-esteem and wellbeing. A great deal of subsequent self-development work through books, various forms of therapy and training, and study and solitude, led her not only to rediscover her confidence but also to find a new peace and a sense of creativity. This has found expression in an exciting new career direction that takes her from her Sydney base to places all around the country.

In her work, Helene draws on her skills in the fields of drama and psychology, her life experiences and her understanding of the wells of both joy and sadness.

If you would like to contact the author, write to Laughter Workshops, PO Box 575, Coogee NSW 2034.

Foreword

Have you ever suffered from 'humouroids'? Humouroids are, by the way, *a hardening of the attitudes which causes piles of problems*!

Just as when we forget to love, if we forget to laugh often enough we soon begin to experience life as hard, tough, a struggle – something to survive rather than to cherish. It is the spirit of laughter that also animates acts of daily kindness, inspires personal creativity, boosts self-esteem, allows our spirit of play, keeps the mind exercised, and generally encourages us to celebrate the gift of life. Without laughter, the celebration of life soon deteriorates into a test of endurance, a fight, a war.

We promise ourselves that one day, after all our problems have been well and truly resolved, we will laugh again, we will love again, we will open our hearts again. The trick is to laugh now, to live now, to open your heart now. Laughter inspires life! Laugh well and you will be in a better position to live well. And as for love, you will find laughter and love give birth to one another, constantly.

I remember the first time Helene ever wrote to me. I was so thrilled to find another 'holy fool' on the planet who was prepared to shout from the rooftops about the importance of love, laughter, fun, joy and happiness. It takes courage. I am blessed to count Helene as a friend. Her presence is the same as her message: warm, loving, alive and highly mischievous. Her workshops are life-affirming. She reminds me that the spirit of joy within me is available at all times if I wish to exercise it. The more I exercise it, the easier it is to enjoy.

Perhaps the biggest contributory cause of illness, or *dis-ease*, on our planet is the belief that happiness exists outside of us and that it must be worked for, earned and deserved before we can enjoy it. Helene tells us, '*Laugh Aerobics* is about showing you how you can connect with your inborn drive to laugh and to appreciate humour, and as a result create more fun, enjoyment, happiness, pleasure and relaxation for yourself'.

The happiness you experience in the world around you is but a dim reflection of the happiness and joy that lives and plays within. Your source of happiness really *is* within, and Helene will help you to help yourself find it, exercise it, play with it and share it with everyone you meet. By deciding to read this book you are deciding to be happy – thank you, for the world needs more than ever before people who are prepared to share their happiness, their love, their joy, their laughter!

Robert Holden
author of *Laughter, The Best Medicine*

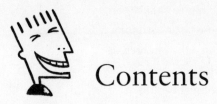

Contents

Considerlafta

Go laughingly, don't worry about where — just go.

Remember what noise there can be in belly-bursters, and as far as possible be on laughing terms even with your enemies: they could teach you a laugh or two.

Speak your jokes only if you can remember the punchline, because even the solemn can out-humour you.

Avoid sad and humourless behaviour: it is a fixation of the serious of spirit.

If you compare yourself to famous comics, keep practising.

Enjoy the fact that your mother laughed at your antics: others may follow her.

Keep interested in your own jokes, even though you've heard them a thousand times.

Exercise copyright if you create good comedy, for the world is full of people looking for one they haven't heard before.

Many persons strive for joy and everywhere there is lightness of humour.

Be you … or find your brand of humour.

Love laughter, for your face will be perennially more youthful.

Take kindly the vernacular of the jocular.

Nurture your sense of humour to shield you in times of sudden stress.

Be full of fun with yourself.

You are a child of the humourverse and as such enjoy the perverse.

Be at peace with the great cosmic chuckle.

It's a funny world and it always offers a bright side, so be funful and laughing.

And don't forget that a daily dose of laughter makes you happy ever after.

Helene Grover

Introduction

Over the years I have become aware that many more people than I can reach through personal contact are interested in my ideas and techniques concerning humour, fun and laughter, and how these can enhance our lives. I received frequent requests for a book that people can read on their own or as an adjunct to coming along to a course or which contains material they can apply informally in a range of settings.

So here is *Laugh Aerobics* – not a philosophical look at laughter but a hands-on one. However it is used, the important thing is to follow the instructions on a sustained basis. I believe that if you do, you can't help but find humour and enjoy life more as a result.

Although I love to laugh and to see others laughing, I'm not a comedian. I'm not much funnier than the next person. I don't aim to amuse through anything I do or say. My approach is: teach people how to laugh, show them that they have the capacity to laugh, and help link them with their own humour. This is the 'difference' I want to make to the world, and the tools I have at my disposal enable me to express and demonstrate the way laughter and humour *can* make a difference.

I am very grateful to all my 'laughter pupils' who have taught me so much. Every time I conduct a seminar, class or workshop, I learn something new. There is always something fresh to realise, new concepts to develop and understandings to reach, other places to go and new audiences to share my discoveries with.

Already I've presented laughter training in many cities, towns and situations. Venues have included schools, halls, private homes, pubs, corporate boardrooms, churches, community centres, clinics, hospitals, staffrooms, nursing homes, healing centres, health retreats, conference centres and festivals.

I've worked with the sad, the fun, the young, the old, the middle-aged, the healthy, the ill, the 'together' and the depleted. Participants have been drawn from many cultures and backgrounds and ways of life. Some of them already know how to enjoy themselves; others admit they have lost their way to fun and joy. A number of them never even began the journey. Sometimes my listeners are resistant and sceptical about the things I suggest to get us going about how healing laughter and humour can be in times of adversity and stress. Others are keen, but self-conscious and inhibited.

It doesn't really matter because once they take part in a session (or even just watch the effect on others), they are won over. I hope that *Laugh Aerobics*, and putting its suggestions in operation, will have the same effect on you. And I hope the awareness and insights you gain will lead to lots of fun and laughter.

1 Born to laugh

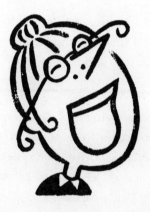

We all want to feel good: healthy, happy, relaxed. And of course what we'd like is to experience these feelings as easily and as often as possible. I've written *Laugh Aerobics* in order to share with you what I know about the quickest, most natural route to feeling good – enjoying plenty of laughter.

Nature uniquely endowed humans with the special capacity for laughter for a reason. And that is, when we laugh we enhance our happiness and wellbeing.

As we shall see, plenty of laughter and fun keeps the body and mind (and, I would argue, the spirit) in far better shape than if we go through life in a solemn and serious way.

Making sure fun and humour feature prominently in our daily lives is just as vital to health as keeping fit and well in other ways. Our day-to day existence – and that of those around us – becomes a lot more enjoyable when we are able to appreciate the lighter side of life (that is always there).

It is increasingly clear that to be fully healthy and to reach their potential, humans need adequate food, water, sleep, exercise, shelter . . . and fun, joy and laughter.

The act of laughing – of 'expressing lively amusement', as the *Concise Oxford Dictionary* refers to it – is not an optional extra, but actually an essential aspect of a successful and satisfying life! Some researchers go as far as to call laughter an instinct. (That's probably a better way of looking at it than to say it's a gift, because a gift implies that while it's a nice thing to have, we don't necessarily need to make use of it.)

If laughter is an instinct, it's something many of us manage to stifle or at least largely lose touch with, especially when we are stressed or when things go wrong. We may know in theory that we like to laugh, but what we need to know in practice is how to do more of it. (I even meet people who fear they've lost the knack completely.) But the good news is that while some people have a greater sense of humour than others – or a better-developed one – we all possess a humorous, fun-loving side. It's just a matter of reconnecting with it, and exercising it!

That's what I help people to do through my laughter-training courses and classes, and what I aim to do through *Laugh Aerobics*. You'll read here about some of the things I suggest my students get up to in workshops in order to provoke fun and laughter, and how you can adapt these ideas for yourself. The cathartic (release of strong emotions) and healing properties of hearty laughter are a fun and gentle way to relieve stress and tension and leave us feeling really good. As we shall see, laughter also has positive effects on creativity and spontaneity.

Benefits long recognised

Throughout the ages – as long ago as ancient Greece and in biblical times – observant people have recognised the beneficial effects of joy and laughter on the mind and body. Their writings are full of accurate comments as to the benefits of fun and mirth on both the well and the sick. In our own more 'scientific' times much of this knowledge has gone unheeded and/or has been discounted. People wanting a 'lift' have been encouraged to take drugs of various kinds to make them feel better rather than being taught about the body's own considerable ability to do this.

But thankfully the tide is turning. The good things that laughter can deliver have become a respectable and important subject of study and research in the United States, Britain and Europe. More and more health professionals, psychologists and researchers are affirming that laughter is stress-relieving and relaxing yet stimulating, as well as having other positive functions. Dozens of books and hundreds of learned papers have now been written detailing the physiological and psychological benefits of laughter. Clinics have even been set up (mostly overseas but a couple in Australia) to promote the role of laughter and humour in health (see Chapter 5).

So what I have to say in *Laugh Aerobics* is not new or radical. What I've done is bring together some material and thoughts that have always been around or have recently been uncovered to do with laughter, and allied them with my own strategies and techniques for bringing it about.

Fit for laughing

Most of us are aware of the need to maintain our physical selves at a reasonable level through a wholesome diet and adequate exercise. For some, the daily routine or playing sport is enough activity to ensure fitness; for others, it is necessary to attend a gym or exercise class or perhaps run, swim or bike-ride to keep in shape.

And some of us neglect our physical fitness to the point that when we do finally exercise, it's a real effort and we're quite surprised how out of form we are. (This is a situation I'm pretty familiar with: too often, when I feel I should be active, to use that apt expression, I lie down until the feeling goes away!)

But just as it's virtually never too late to do something about our bodies, we can also do something about the fun aspect of our lives. When we aim to increase our physical fitness we are prepared to undertake some unaccustomed activities. So it is that there are all sorts of measures we can take to improve our health and contentment through reviving the humorous aspect of our lives.

The reasons why

There are many reasons why laughter is such a good thing to get lots of. We don't need experts to tell us what many of them are, but all the same it's fascinating to hear about what benefits have now been 'officially' recognised. Here are some of them. (There will be more in years to come; there's much yet that is still to be learned about the subject.)

- By distracting us from worry and gloomy thoughts, if only for a few moments, laughing can lighten stress, anxiety, depression and pain. Laughter relaxes the body and the mind, at the same time leaving us stimulated. Or as one American professor puts it, 'Laughter is stressful in the way a passionate kiss is: it excites us and makes us feel great'.

- When we laugh we are in the present, here and now, even if laughing about previous events. When we are in the happy present, the past and future recede and cease to bother us. The more the laughter, the longer lasting is the effect.

- Laughter gives a hearty work-out to practically every organ in the body. This is really great news. Norman Cousins (see pages 119–22) coined the term 'internal jogging' for laughing, and I think it's a terrific one.

  (The term 'internal jogging' is appropriate because laughing provides the body with a cardiovascular work-out, hence the title of this book. When we laugh, our heart rate and blood pressure rise, getting the circulation going. When we've finished laughing, they drop to pre-laugh levels, leaving us feeling relaxed and refreshed.)

- Another effect of laughter is to cause our lungs to rapidly inhale and exhale and our muscles to let go of tension as they contract and then relax. (Get into a good laugh and the muscles of your arms and legs will be involved as well.) That's why we feel pleasantly 'saggy' afterwards and our diaphragm and abdomen can ache for a short while.

- When we laugh we activate the production of a range of hormones (substances produced by the endocrine system which regulate specific actions in our cells and organs) which do various systems in the body a great deal of good. For example, laughter releases endorphins and enkephalins – which are natural painkillers – and puts us in a good mood. (The so-called 'runner's high' is due to the same effect.)

- The connection between the mind and the body is so strong that laughter causes the brain to pour out chemicals that balance left- and right-brain activity. This balance enhances and increases our creative capacities and leads to clearer thinking and alertness. (You can read more about the link between laughter and creativity on pages 46–48.)

- It is very important to our health that we maintain a strong immune system that can deal effectively with viruses, bacteria and malignant cells. In an interesting experiment carried out in the United States that showed the effect of laughter on this front-line defence, the levels of subjects' immune proteins increased dramatically after they watched a comic film. Remarkably, they stayed at this high level even when the group subsequently watched serious films. Other evidence also points to the fact that the experience of humour boosts levels of immunoglobulin A, a virus-fighter found in saliva.

- Researchers have discovered that among the hormones released by laughter are catecholamines, which have anti-inflammatory properties. This has implications for those living with arthritis and other inflammatory conditions.
- There is evidence that laughter could be therapeutic for high blood pressure through sustained arterial relaxation that improves the flow of blood.

There are some very serious people going about evaluating the business of laughter. When a journal as prestigious and conservative as that of the American Medical Association admits that 'A humour therapy group can improve the quality of life for patients with chronic problems. Laughter has immediate symptom-relieving effects for those patients', you can be sure they've undertaken a thorough investigation before making such a statement.

We make ourselves laugh

Before we go any further, there is something I must get straight. I don't try to make people laugh! I mention this early on because the misconception often arises.

In the workshops, seminars and classes I organise myself, I explain to my listeners why I'm there. But when I give talks and presentations to, say, work groups or in institutions, I am usually introduced by someone else. So often this person says to the audience, 'This is Helene Grover, she runs laughter workshops and she is now going to make us laugh'. My heart sinks!

I then have to explain that this is not what I am about to do at all. Making people laugh is not my business; I don't want that role and that responsibility. Besides, terrific though laughing is, if I merely made people laugh, that would be the beginning and the end of it.

Making people laugh is the role of a comic, comedian, clown, humorist, actor, magician and others who entertain by their antics, either verbal or physical. All the audience has to do is sit and watch or listen and choose whether to laugh or not to laugh at the performer.

None of the above roles are mine. My role is to show people how whether they laugh or not is a choice; to raise awareness that we choose whether or not to be amused by whatever happens. Nothing is preordained as funny; just about anything has the potential to amuse us if we choose to see it that way.

What I aim to achieve is longer-term: to show that each of us is responsible for ourselves, for our own feelings and actions, and for our reactions to what happens to us. Following on from that we are also responsible for our own joy and our own humour. No one can actually 'make' you laugh. My hope is that I help you become aware of your capacity for humour and create an awareness that there are many things to laugh about.

The ideas you'll read about here I've developed over the years in the 'laughter-training' workshops I conduct around Australia and through the many talks and seminars on the value of laughter that I've given. The purpose of these activities is to encourage people to examine their beliefs about laughter and their backgrounds in relation to laughter, fun and humour, and to identify what may be holding them back from enjoying more.

In my workshops we do all sorts of things to encourage laughter, have some fun, be less inhibited, loosen up – whatever you want to call it. Nothing is forced, participants join in at their own level – which may be just to sit and watch.

When people experience how good it feels to let go and laugh (or observe others doing so) and then try out my techniques and ideas in their own time on a regular basis, the benefits can start to come very quickly.

A typical experience

I see many examples of change when people start to emphasise fun in their daily lives rather than tension and gloom. The turn-around in George, a participant in one of my workshops who learnt to value and create his own humour, is typical.

In our first group session we talked about how you can take your mind away from stressful situations by introducing some silly or fun element. As homework, I asked participants to make a laughter or fun commitment for the week.

The following session George reported: 'I've had the most amazing time! I consciously set out to see the funny side of things and it worked! I tuned in to a whole new spectrum of humour . . . Suddenly I noticed the lack of humour in my environment and what that did to people.

'During the week I had to conduct some difficult job interviews and the way I dealt with them, applying the techniques you taught, made them much easier and lighter and personally less stressful. Most of the stress in the past, I realised, had come from the way I was thinking'.

The same principles apply to those intending to try these ideas for themselves. Certainly in a group helpful dynamics can apply, but there's no reason why you can't successfully follow the instructions in this book in your own time, on your own ground. (After a while you'll probably find yourself putting more effort into seeking out groups of people you enjoy being with because you'll come to treasure the laughs you have together.)

Learn to laugh from a book?

But can a book show you how to laugh, or laugh more? I get asked this question a lot. On the surface it does seem a rather strange thing, especially as *Laugh Aerobics* doesn't in itself contain humour or anything necessarily intended to amuse you.

The way I see it, *Laugh Aerobics* is in some respects like a book you might read in order to enhance your sex life. Such a book would look at the physical and emotional dimensions of the situation, outline some techniques and strategies to improve matters, recommend some things to practise and consider incorporating into everyday life. It's up to you to try them out and adapt them according to your tastes. So it is with laughter.

But although reading about either of these enjoyable aspects of life can be useful as a guide, the rewards come only when you try out on a sustained basis what works for you. (Here my parallels with sex end. Unlike that other fun activity, with laughter you don't have to undress or prepare: you just get into the experience – anywhere, in any position; you feel good afterwards.)

Laughter and sex do share a parallel, though, in the area of vulnerability. In certain situations, sex can make us feel vulnerable and so – for different reasons – can laughter. For some people, expressing laughter or creating some fun means stepping out of their comfort zone. The very thought can make them uncomfortable: 'What will others think if I laugh right now?' and 'I have a peculiar laugh' are common reactions. Laughing is often done publicly and among strangers and we can't be sure of the effect it will have on others. I hear more from people about the possible embarrassment of laughing than about anything else, about the embarrassment of laughing when no one else does.

I tell them I understand how they feel, but I beg them not to let these feelings stifle a laugh or stop their having some fun. 'If you feel that something is funny', I tell them, 'even if you are the only one of this opinion, go ahead and laugh. Don't miss out on it!' Bringing down the barriers, stretching the comfort zone a little, are what it's all about.

So yes, in some instances laughter may make you vulnerable, but so does breathing . . .

Connecting with your humour

Laugh Aerobics is about showing you how you can connect with your inborn drive to laugh and to appreciate humour, and as a result create more fun, enjoyment, happiness, pleasure and relaxation for yourself.

Fundamental to this, of course, is the recognition that everyone finds different things to laugh at and about: each sense of humour is individual, each funny bone is tickled in different ways. My methods for identifying humorous and/or laughter-creating situations are intended as a springboard for you to discover what works best for you personally.

(Although they are both mechanisms for coping with many stressors in our lives, humour is not always accompanied by laughter. Humour involves detaching ourselves from a situation in order to recognise what amuses us – which we may appreciate inwardly or outwardly – while laughter is more a physiological response to a range of triggers. I don't want to provide a definition here: I want to point out the basic difference.)

Humour is the way you view the world, the way you perceive what goes into your mind and the recognition of, as one writer has put it, 'perceiving some comedy in our chaos'. But an appreciation of humour is not just luck; it can also be a specifically learned skill. Developing this skill means you can deal with change more flexibly, be creative under pressure, work better, play more enjoyably and become healthier in the process. But the skill has to be practised until it becomes part of you and the way you live. Then, when you need the benefits of humour the most, you have the ability to make use of it to communicate, to let off steam, to cope with difficult situations.

Underlying all I have to say is the desirability of cultivating something very important and valuable, which life isn't much fun without – humour awareness. What humour awareness means is always being at the ready to pick up on, and respond to, anything that strikes you as worthy of enjoyment.

Humour is all around us, we just have to tune in to it. I've found it helpful in my own life and in working with students to imagine picking up on humour with an imaginary device I call a humour radar.

Think of it rather like an antenna jutting out of the top of your head. Constantly searching for laughter material, it finds anything around you that's funny, fun, worth writing down, worth telling others about, worth remembering, worth having a go at.

The antenna isn't only working to provide big belly laughs, the things you're going to recall and chuckle about in a month's time. It works just as well for the quick smile in response to something passingly amusing, a bit of a giggle at something you forget a minute later. Lots of smaller appreciations of humour a day are just as useful as a few big ones, especially if the latter are difficult to come by. (People who laugh easily and a lot don't hold themselves back waiting for something really funny to occur: they let themselves be amused by a whole range of things along the way.)

A well-functioning antenna will also focus on yourself, identifying the funny things you do, say, think, feel, and reflecting your humour back to you so you can enjoy it. It's not only others who provide material for laughter; it's also your own interactions, the thoughts that come to you when alone, and the ironies, incongruities and paradoxes of life.

The more your antenna has to work with, the more it comes up with. The more funny things it locates, the better you feel. You will discover humour alone or with others, in your home, at work, during leisure pursuits, in the backyard, in the countryside, in the city. It doesn't matter where or with whom, because the recognition and enjoyment of the joke comes from within yourself.

Humour awareness

I try as much as possible to keep my humour antenna up. This can be a challenge when I'm preoccupied with other things or I'm going through a particularly difficult time. Here are a couple of small and unintentional examples of humour which gave me a good chuckle and which I recall with private pleasure . . .

I was browsing in a Jewish bookshop not long ago when two young men came in and tried to sell the elderly owner (who wore a yarmulke – a skullcap – which indicated he was a religious man) some bags. Oblivious to their surroundings, they'd tried to persuade him he should get some in stock for Christmas. I couldn't help overhearing and couldn't help laughing at the absurdity of it all.

I said to the young men, 'This is really funny. Do you guys know where you are?'

'Oh, you can sell these bags in any shop', they said. 'They're okay for a bookshop, too.'

'This is a Jewish bookshop', I replied. 'We don't have Christmas.'

'It doesn't matter, lady', came the quick response. 'These bags would make a great gift!'

By this time a couple of other people had come in but no one except me saw the humour. However, because of my amusement the owner said 'You look like a good laugher, I'll tell you a couple of things', and he went on to relate some truly funny stories. I went home feeling uplifted and pleased about our connection.

The other story concerns my desexed male German shepherd dog in which a little terrier was recently showing a great deal of interest. The pest followed us on our walk, constantly trying to get intimately close to my dog. When I began to shoo it away, it tried to ingratiate itself with me and started licking my hand. I was in the middle of saying 'Now look here you randy little thing, this is no way to behave', when a couple of people passed by, giving me some very quizzical looks! Then they stopped, clicked to what was going on and laughed with me. We all went on our way, cheered by our unexpected sharing of humour.

Court jesters, a feature of courts in medieval times and before, were not just men dressed up in funny costumes. They had a definite job to do. Through jokes, silly antics and amusing comments, their task was to make the king and those around him forget their worries and indulge in a good laugh. Even back then it was realised that with laughter and fun comes a restoration of physical and emotional wellbeing.

Native Americans were on to something too. Raymond Moody (see page 117) tells how many tribes had orders of ceremonial 'clowns' who, through 'weird dress and outrageous behaviour', provoked laughter in others. Laughter was known to be health-giving.

This doesn't sound too different from the circus clowns of today or the reason behind the introduction of clowns into the wards of some children's hospitals. What a pity today we consider ourselves so 'sophisticated' that their zany antics are mostly seen as appropriate only for the young.

Laugh aerobics

So many people these days go to aerobic exercise classes or to a gym or get fit at home or through other efforts of their own that the word 'aerobics' has become part of our everyday language.

The kind of aerobics this book suggests is to do with getting your sense of humour into shape. As I've already admitted, I'm not big on physical exercise but for the sake of my health I make sure I give myself a laughter work-out very often. This is in addition to the laughs that I pick up on as often as possible.

Aerobics and any kind of physical exercise that gives you a good cardiovascular work-out releases natural endorphins in the body. This is why we feel good after a bout of vigorous activity. Laughing heartily also releases endorphins. By combining activity and laughter – laugh aerobics – we receive a double dose!

What I call 'laugh aerobics' is unique to my workshops and to my way of working with laughter. Laugh aerobics is a set of techniques and exercises you can perform to get the laughter going, and also to act as a catalyst for creating your own variations. You can do them by yourself or apply them to settings such as a workplace, a voluntary organisation, a community group (for example, a youth group, a mothers' group, an unemployment group, a self-help group), within the family, in the classroom, on a group outing, before a meeting, at a sporting club and so on. Although group laughter is contagious, the ultimate effect of this fun energiser is the same no matter how many people are involved.

Once you start the laughter juices flowing with some laugh aerobics, you're set for finding other things to laugh at.

'Tee hee, Ha ha' *Actually*

Here is a basic exercise, which is fun and effective, to get you going. I teach this 'Tee hee, Ha ha' work-out in the first session of a course and we do it again each week. I also recommend that participants do it between meetings at home and keep up the practice after the course has finished. The idea is to make a lot of noise out of the sounds we use for laughter and to throw your limbs and trunk vigorously into the movements as if you were doing aerobics. (Of course, if this part is difficult for you, do the exercise at a level you are comfortable with.)

Quickly raise your arms, one at a time, above your head and punch the air shouting 'Tee hee' with abandon. Return your arms quickly to your sides. Now throw your arms up to shoulder level and shout 'Ha ha'. Then put your hands on your hips, turn your torso to the right and shout 'Hee hee', then to the left, making the same sound. You could also fling your hips to the right and left in the movement. Now lower your arms, immediately raising your knees one at a time, slapping each and saying 'Ho ho'. Finish by pressing your finger on top of your head, pirouetting as you say 'Tee hee, Ha ha, Hee hee, Ho ho'.

Keep going briskly with these or similar movements, accompanying them with any other fun sounds you can come up with. Go faster or slower as you fancy, but obviously you get a better work-out if you do the exercise quickly and loudly. As with all my suggestions, the aim is not to 'get it right' but to 'get it fun' (see pages 104–05).

Sometimes I do a version in my car (car aerobics) when I want to prevent myself getting stressed at bad drivers. Doing silly things inside the car keeps me engaged and amused at my own antics, which means that I can't be engaged with aggravation and aggression.

If you'd like to try the idea, remember to keep your hands on the wheel at all times and your eyes on the road (or wait until you are stopped, when you can remove one or both hands). The idea is to use your fingers to make silly little movements or put a silly look on your face, and at the same time mutter or shout quickly some crazy syllables – Tee hee, Ha ha, Ho ho, Knik knik, Moo moo – whatever you like. Again, it sounds silly written down. Again, it works.

As the brain can only cope with one thing at a time, laugh aerobics like these give it a rest, some time out. Use them to provide the brain with a break or to get it started in a new direction.

Turn to Chapter 3 for more laugh aerobics you can use in different situations.

Sometimes people say to me that they would like to laugh more and get more fun out of life but they haven't got anything to laugh about or they are not in the mood.

Waiting until you are in the mood to laugh could take a long time, I tell them. To wait until you feel like laughing is to put the cart before the horse. Laugh first, I advise, and that will put you in the mood. Just like the saying 'Appetite comes with eating', laughter comes from laughing.

Laugh despite the traumas

This is not to suggest that you bury the traumas of your life under a rug and pretend that stresses don't exist, nor that you live in a state of denial and keep smiling when you are feeling a lot of pain. What I'm advocating is to look honestly at what's bothering you, to seek therapeutic or other help if that's appropriate and, in addition, to cultivate a positive stance helped along by ensuring that you bring some humour to it. It will really lighten the load.

I recall giving a talk to a group of elderly people who were pretty negative and unenthusiastic about whatever I said. They came from the same cultural background as myself, so I realised I would need to tap in to that to get the best out of them.

'So, what did you expect from me today?' I asked them.

A variety of voices replied, 'We want jokes. Isn't that what you are going to do, make us laugh?'

'No', I answered. 'If that's what you think, I'm going home. Bye!' I pretended to walk off.

'No, no, don't go', they said. 'We heard you were terrific, and seeing you're here why don't you stay?'

I was halfway there. I judged they were ready for me to start talking again about the importance of laughter, but all I could see were frown lines deep enough to plant banana trees in. So I said, 'I suppose you think you've got nothing to laugh about?' The roomful of faces nodded. 'I suppose you think you're too sick?' More nods. 'I imagine you're upset that you don't see enough of your children and grandchildren?' Vigorous nodding. 'I can also understand that you may have some financial difficulties?' Another round of assent.

'Life is just too difficult right now for you to get up to this nonsense, isn't that so?' Most people were by now not only nodding but also smiling that I should be so clever as to know what they were thinking. (In any presentation it is vital to let your listeners know that you understand and that you are just another person with problems like them, not someone who has all the answers . . . Just some of them!)

The rest of the talk seemed to be received in a mixed fashion. However, at the end I got lots of questions, applause and hugs from members of the audience. They told me I was the most successful speaker they'd ever had. This was a big surprise. 'Oh, believe us, you were successful. You know why? You were the first speaker that no one fell asleep on! We were all wide awake.'

'Put on a happy face' is not just a line from a song. Putting on a face is worth remembering to do each day for the reason that it does you good all over. When you smile, the tightening of the facial muscles alters the blood flow in the head and decreases the temperature of the blood supply to the brain. This is associated with feeling good. The great thing is the smile or the laugh doesn't even have to be genuine: your body and brain can't tell the difference between a fake laugh and a real one!

Fake laughter produces the same chemicals in the brain as real laughter. So 'fake it till you make it' when you need to create an instant laugh to help you cope with stress, pain or being stuck in gloom. A fake laugh, you'll find, has the potential to bring on the real thing. It's also a valuable tactic for those who have trouble with the physical act of laughing. So until you find it easy to get your laughter quotient through humour, just pretend!

Laughing matters

Laughter, I admit, appears to come more easily to some people than to others. There are those who seem to have been born with a bubbling sense of humour, a capacity to be readily amused, the ability to see the funny side of even adverse circumstances. Some of these people not only like to observe fun but they also make it happen.

Then there are those who laugh when something strikes them as particularly funny, but it may be some time between laughs and they do little to create them. The remainder are even harder to move to mirth; they may have been conditioned against it or their personality may tend to view life from a more serious, unspontaneous perspective . . . Not a laughing matter.

Whichever category you identify with (and you may move between them at times), I believe that if you really want to enjoy more laughs and bring more fun into your life, you can develop your ability to do so. Indeed, a favourite saying of my American mentor and teacher in the field of laughter, Dr Annette Goodheart, comes from philosopher William James: 'We don't laugh because we're happy, we're happy because we laugh'.

Like me, you're probably amazed at the number of books available that aim to show you how to have a happier, more satisfying and productive life. Much of what they advocate is absolutely spot-on – if you can do it.

Sound in theory as they may be, the majority of these books require such solid work to be put into practice that most of them are probably never read right through, let alone acted on. This is because they require you to transform yourself through conscious effort, and that's an enormous challenge. When you've put a lot of effort into working through your problems, faced what's causing you trouble and changed your attitudes, you'll feel better, they claim . . . But it could take a long time.

Some of what I advocate in *Laugh Aerobics* can work pretty well instantaneously. This is not because you have to resolve your problems or stresses or your future before you can enjoy life, but because laughter can instantly cause us to feel better. When we laugh we take some 'time out' from worrying or being caught in a downward spiral. A good bout of laughter interrupts the panic/pain cycle of our thought processes, gives our brains a jolt and releases the 'happy hormones' that make us feel better.

You can do it

Whenever I'm moaning and groaning about my life for some reason, and then I stop and recognise that if I want it to be better then I'm the only one who can wave the magic wand and change my perspective, that's when the most exciting and positive things have happened. It's these perspective-changing techniques that I aim to convey through *Laugh Aerobics*.

Even if much of what is written here serves to show you how far you have to go to cultivate a more fun approach to life (attending a workshop often engenders the same reaction), that knowledge in itself is valuable. The seed has been planted and won't be smothered again.

2 Focus on fun

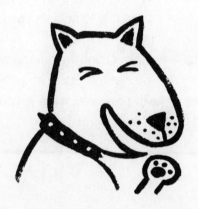

So powerful is the thinking process that we can create virtually anything in our minds (as we will see when we look later at how attitudes colour our thoughts and our world). What is at work here is our imagination . . . which we can use either for or against ourselves.

Although our imagination is working hard all the time, we may need to train it to work differently to create the sort of environment we like and want, an environment that includes plenty of fun and laughter. When we stop using our imagination to come up with negatives and start using it to produce some positive images and attitudes, good things begin to happen.

Deep inside us all there is something akin to, in effect, a magic wand. That's what I call it anyway. Others refer to this concept of our power to create our own world by other terms such as a 'higher self'. The name doesn't matter, though I find the idea of a magic wand a colourful and graphic one. Indeed it is sometimes used, literally and figuratively, in therapy.

With the thought of a wand in our mind we can create our own joy and happiness. Visualise this device and use your imagination to see it waving over you, making you feel good in mind and body.

Our playful selves

One of the things that happens when we let our imagination and creativity run free is that we release our playful selves. This playful part of ourselves is just one of the many facets of who we are.

We all play a multitude of roles in life, assuming different ones at different times in order to deal with the varying situations in which we find ourselves. Think of all the facets of you that are probably called on every day: citizen, partner, worker, parent, grandparent, consumer, commuter, neighbour, son, daughter, householder and so on. They all go to make us who we are. The playful self is in there too, and can play a part in all these roles.

Our playful self (which comes from the concept of playful child-within) is to do with fun and spontaneity and naturalness, of finding delight in life and in small things the way children do as they discover the world. Children know how to play; they don't have to be taught. They don't question why something is fun, they just do it for its own sake without inhibition or judgement. If you wish to be closer to children – yours or others' – join them in play. Children love grown-ups who know how to have fun and how to play, especially with them.

The forgotten self

One of my aims is to help people release their playful selves in all aspects of life. Often participants in my workshops go on to discover that they were never really playful when they were children. Their early life may have hurt and repressed them and they may not have been encouraged to play and have fun; they may have had to grow up too fast.

I can identify with that in my own life. I was born during the Second World War when life was a matter of survival. My parents had little time, opportunity or inclination to play with me and no means to buy me toys. Later on, I still didn't catch up. I was ten when my father died and I had to take care of business for my mother and myself.

If it has been hard for me to connect with who I can really be, how much more so for people who were abused or neglected as children or for whom other things have robbed them of their natural childhood? In my workshops I've had the opportunity to observe just how far some people's playful sides have been pushed away, and how sturdy are the walls they have erected around themselves. Those protective mechanisms served to protect the playful self during the period of danger, but now the time has come for that aspect to emerge and make up for lost opportunities. This is the challenge.

How many readers can identify with a childhood that held taboos about noise and spontaneity, that suppressed exuberance and playfulness? I hear a fair bit about the blocking of this sort of natural fun, and also about the curbing messages from adults – 'Be quiet', 'Stop that silly behaviour' and 'You're giving me a headache' – and the effect they had.

So many childhood messages had to do with putting aside play until we had completed the things we had to do. Now we are adults ourselves we can make our own choices. Where we choose to bring play into our activities (including work) we actually increase our creativity, positivity and learning capacity.

Grab the humour that presents itself even in unpromising circumstances because it can get us through some bad spots and add to the good ones. For example, not long ago I was on my way to give a laughter seminar at the hospital where my mother had died. I had not been back since and was feeling pretty uptight.

Then, when I was stopped at traffic lights, I saw a man and a woman walking their dogs. His was a sleek chihuahua and hers was a fluffy silky-haired terrier, and I immediately thought, '"His" and "Hers" dogs!'. This made me laugh and I kept the image for a while as I drove along. It was enough to give me the coping trigger I needed to face the seminar.

Laughter and tears

One of my early workshops taught me a lot about the vulnerability of the playful child. I was focused on laughter, watching participants have fun using the toys I had brought along (I often use toys as an aid in accessing the fun aspect of us, see pages 39–42) and testing out some techniques for humour. While I was prepared for some people to be shy or to think my ideas were too silly for them to try, I was not equipped to deal with crying.

The tears came from a woman who just sat to one side of the room. At the time I was not as well equipped to deal with occurrences such as crying. A lot of training, reading and the development of awareness has led me to the understanding that when you work with and about laughter, you can also bring about tears. Laughter can be the other side of tears and sometimes the two reactions can be very close to one another. (For those who work in this area, it is vital to recognise this fact and to develop the skills to perceive it and deal with it. Techniques for dealing with situations in which painful feelings are brought to the surface are a must. In this respect, I have a lot of time for the writings of John Bradshaw, who works so extensively with boundary setting and healing the wounded inner child.)

Over the years I've seen too many workshop leaders and facilitators work with people on an emotional level but not be sensitive to the needs of those they are dealing with. Many self-awareness processes are very confronting in one way or another, even in laughter (and in reading a book like this) and they can leave people feeling exposed and vulnerable. There can be many issues and hidden agendas attached to laughter and while people come along to sessions in order to lighten up, to find their sense of humour, fun and laughter, they bring with them the very constrictions that blocked them from that in the first place.

When we reached the 'playful self' segment, the woman cried some more. Obviously what we were doing had touched a deep chord. At the end of the session I advised her to try to identify whatever it was that led her to release the tears and if necessary to phone me to talk about it.

She did, the next day. She told me that as a child her mother would stand over her with her fist ready to hit her every time she made a noise or laughed. To her, laughter represented pain. No wonder sadness came to the fore in the class and that she needed to work through repressed pain before she could connect with the laughter she also possessed.

This woman had attended the workshop, she said, because she had had enough of being serious and she wanted to learn how to give herself permission to start enjoying herself. I suggested she ease into this by buying a teddy bear, nurturing herself for a while, and then starting to make laughter sounds like 'Tee hee, Ha ha' (see pages 18–19), giving herself permission to come out and play. This way she would learn as an adult it was okay to laugh, to have fun, to be spontaneous, to make a noise. I also suggested she continue therapy.

I didn't hear from her again but as she had already made a breach in the barriers she'd understandably built up around herself, I was sure that in due course she'd pull down the rest, too.

Finding fun

Our society is so based on achievement, on setting and reaching goals, on being the best, on winning, that we often neglect to have fun along the way. Just for a change, for the sake of laughter and spontaneity, do what you have to do – the fun way. If it's not the right way, laugh about it and enjoy the things that come up as you take an alternative path.

Unfortunately, rigid people often tend to take the creation of laughter and play as seriously as they take other tasks. They practise my techniques in a serious fashion, really only doing them because I told them to. They need to learn to have fun learning to have fun!

It's best not to judge what is fun: your idea will be different from mine, which will be different from other people's. Fun is whatever you think it is and wherever you find it. It can lie in the unexpected, the unusual, the unlikely, the unpredictable. So don't limit yourself by deciding in advance what is fun and what is not. Be prepared to be surprised – by yourself! You will also find that other people's idea of fun can also be worth exploring . . . Give it a go!

Don't leave fun to chance

Here are some techniques for getting you going. Remember
that having fun doesn't have to cost anything or be difficult
to organise or even involve others.

First, make a list of all the things you find fun to do; it
doesn't matter if they are accessible or possible right now,
just start the list. Do it for yourself, not for what you think
others will approve of. Stick the list up on a wall or the fridge
and keep adding ideas for fun to it.

Once you've been working on this list for a time, start a
second list, the fun enquiry list. Ask everyone you know what
they think is fun. They'll come up with things you hadn't
considered and you'll find lots of inspiration through hearing
their ideas. (You'll also find that talking about such topics leads
to closer communication with all sorts of people, from those
you know well to those you don't.)

Now start thinking about the fun things you can do while
you're doing something else, and make another list. Note the
everyday activities you already do, like going for a walk or
watching TV or changing nappies or washing the dishes, and
work out how you can add a fun dimension. For example,
don't limit yourself to just 'doing' things; add 'thinking' and
'feeling' things as well. You could sing mock opera style
about what you are doing, you could do a running com-
mentary as if you were describing the activity on radio, you
could imagine you were being filmed or that you are a particular cartoon character or comedian and so on.

Now look again at all your lists and mark the fun things
you can get under way immediately and the ones that will
have to wait a bit (although try not to put things off: we miss

out on a lot of fun by deferring it). Add some dates for the fun things you plan, no matter how small. Try to plan something minor for each day, then something bigger for each week, then a major fun event once a month. This doesn't have to be big or expensive. It could be going to a funny movie, to a fun park, to theatre sports or to something else that makes you laugh. It could be going on a picnic or a short trip, following up an interest, seeing someone who cheers you up. I also recommend playing with toys and games . . . Why should children have all the fun?

If you fear others making fun of you for any reason – minor mishaps, a disadvantage, a disability, something you feel uncomfortable about – find a way for others to laugh with you. This is a challenge for creating some self-humour. This is different from putting yourself down, which you should never do.

You can sometimes make yourself and others laugh by telling the simple truth. When people expect you to have the answers, especially if you usually do, the unexpectedness of your saying casually 'Gosh, I don't know', can bring a guffaw of surprise. You can even manage here to look quite pleased with yourself! (If you examine humorous situations, you'll often find that a common ingredient is that of surprise.)

Some low-cost, fun examples

The couple of free or low-cost activities I typically incorporate in my own life show how laughter is potentially found everywhere, even in unlikely settings. Humour is indeed in the mind of the beholder.

One of my most enjoyable activities is to take a walk on the beach near my home. I love to watch the seagulls: they can be very funny. They strut around, throw tantrums, screech and fight. They certainly don't share. I often have a laugh at their antics and sometimes have been joined by children on the beach and we've laughed together.

Another spontaneous happening that I value in my memory and in the retelling, also occurred close to home. I like to enjoy a coffee with a friend at a nearby seaside hotel. We sit over our cups in the foyer for ages, watching the passing parade. It never disappoints. This particular day a wedding, a football team and a fancy-dress party swirled around us!

First came the bride and flower girl, followed by the wedding guests with bunches of white balloons, then people dressed in wild-west costumes. They were followed by a team of American rugby players. At the same time a couple of the bridesmaids from the wedding started having an argument, then one of the guests tried to chat one of them up. Along came a man in a dinner suit juggling three oranges, then a short person with some coloured balloons, then Uncle Sam accompanied by an astronaut and Colonel Sanders. It was the best free entertainment we could have had.

Even where the people who pass you by are not very interesting or eye-catching in themselves, you can still have fun making up stories about them or hypothesising about what would happen if . . .

Remind yourself to lighten up

There are many fun things you can tap into that are not difficult to arrange, that are cheap and can be done on your own. In themselves they are tiny, but the effect is cumulative. Some are funny in themselves, others will remind you to lighten up:

- Place some smiley-face stickers around your home and workplace. On your phone or computer are good spots, as is on the letterbox. Clown or fairy stickers are fun too.
- Put a plastic mouse on your cheese platter.
- Paint a smiley face on your big toe.
- Decide to have a great day.
- Fly a kite.
- Take some children to the zoo and mimic the animals.
- Read humorous cards in shops.
- Buy a parrot or budgie and teach it to say 'A laugh a day', 'Go on, laugh', 'Tee hee' or whatever takes your fancy. (Even a battery-operated bird can be fun to have around.)
- Learn to see and hear laughter in everything. A brook babbles and also laughs; birds sing and also laugh!
- Canned laughter on televison is good for bringing on laughter. Be part of that response – natural or contrived. Laugh along; picture yourself as a light-hearted person, laughing.
- Even if you believe you're not in the mood to laugh, feel your muscles relax as you smile. Lift the corners of your

mouth into a gentle smile and keep smiling. Feel the muscles of your body relax. Turning on a smile – even one that doesn't have a basis at that point in humour – repels tensions produced by stress. A smile is halfway to a healthy laugh. If you go on to laugh, you'll release even more tension.

- Delight in funny sounds, as children do at the blurt of a tuba, the crash of a cymbal, the thump of a big drum. Listen for new and funny noises that can make you laugh.
- Have a truly-me day or half day where you only do things that please you and when you are aware of only good things around you.
- If you live on your own or with someone who is difficult and not in tune with humour, make sure you stay focused on your right to create your own laughs and indulge in your own brand of fun.

Whether something is silly or not is usually a matter of opinion. If the thought of being silly gives you problems, change the label you give an activity or idea and suddenly it will seem valid (especially if you tell yourself it's good for you). Being silly is not being stupid, by the way. 'Stupid' implies that you did something because you didn't know any better or you made a foolish choice; 'silly', which derives from an Old English word meaning both happy and blessed, refers to fun and nonsense that you choose to indulge in for enjoyment.

Go away and play

I never cease to be surprised with what people in my laughter-training classes come up with when they go home with the instructions to make sure they have fun during the coming week. The following accounts are real examples of what some people did. They might trigger off an idea for a bit of everyday fun of your own.

- Mick went to the live taping of a favourite comedy show on TV. Given the group dynamics, being part of the studio audience made for a much funnier experience than watching the show at home, he reported.

- Michelle played a fun game with her flatmates. They tied balloons to their ankles and then tried to pop each other's balloons. The last person to have an unpopped balloon won. Sounds like something kids would do – but so what? It generated a lot of laughter. (Laughter combined with a physical activity such as this is super-good for relieving stress and inducing feelings of relaxation.)

- Denise created some domestic humour that we all enjoyed hearing about: 'Our house has a plague of lost socks; it's a real nuisance. So I found a piece of driftwood and placed over it all the single lost socks lying around the place. I set my children a competition, telling them that I would give them a sweet for each sock they found that would make up a matching pair with one on the wood. It really worked and gave us a lot of family fun.

  'I also ran a sock-of-the-month competition. The winner was a well-worn red sock on which I then sewed buttons for eyes and a mouth. I brought it to the laughter class and used it as a hand puppet. So I got a lot of mileage out of a bit of nonsense'.

- Helen told us she is a naturally outrageous person. She used this to her advantage by threatening her children – who are sometimes concerned about how far Mum will go – that she would do something outrageous if they didn't behave! (It worked.)

In my workshops one of the first things I do is ask participants what they find funny, what appeals to their particular sense of humour. This is not just an empty query. Replying gives us all the chance to open up to each other a little and provides lots of ideas for increasing our own breadth of enjoyment. People come up with all sorts of answers that the rest of us hadn't necessarily considered. (This is the way I came to appreciate Mr Bean! It has also led to my collecting those wonderful notices for travellers posted in fractured English in overseas hotels. They never fail to give me a giggle.)

You can copy this idea in your own life, asking others about their humour or just observing the humour they enjoy. You may find you've been restricting your ability to look for laughs by rejecting certain avenues or by not knowing about some sources.

While it may not seem very spontaneous to plan deliberately to have fun, if you start putting your plans into action you'll find that it all becomes natural and spontaneous quite quickly. You'll realise that you are feeling good, that you are getting a whole lot more of what you want, that you are achieving things you did not think you could and that you are less stressed. This is good news if you're a 'recovering serious person'. (This phrase was coined by a laughter-training colleague of mine in the United States. He once said he was a recovering alcoholic and so came up with 'recovering serious person'. I really like the term.)

Toys are not just for kids

As I have pointed out earlier, we can learn so much from children, to whom having fun, laughing and playing are the stuff of life. One of the things fundamental to their lives is toys. I've made toys part of mine too (to great benefit). I take toys and fun gadgets to my workshops to give participants the opportunity to have fun with them and to give them ideas for buying a toy of their own. It's amazing how many people have incorporated toys in their daily lives and what it achieves for them. Sometimes it acts simply as a reminder to have fun.

So do yourself a favour and buy yourself a toy! Do what children do and look at lots, deciding what appeals, and choose one you really would like to have around to play with.

If you haven't already done so, acquiring a teddy bear is a good idea. Teddies have many uses: from something to hug, nurture or talk to, all the way to healing. Hugging reconnects us with the sense of touch and takes us straight into the child's world. (For therapists working with abused children, touching is obviously a very sensitive issue. Teddy bears are often used in these situations to introduce children to the idea that touching and being touched can be safe and pleasant.)

In the past, my living space had no toys or fun things in it. Since I've started to work in the field of laughter, my house looks rather different, partly because I've bought items to take to seminars and partly because I now enjoy having fun things around. I'm aware that I'm making up for lost opportunities when I was a child . . . And that's fine.

I have a toy parrot that, when you press a button, repeats what you say (fun at a dinner party); a smiley soft toy; pepper and salt shakers that say 'Ah-choo' and 'Bless you' when shaken; a clown puppet on a string. I don't have so many things that the house looks like a child-minding centre, but I have just enough bits and pieces to remind me that fun and nonsense are as important as anything else in life.

An important component of my workshops is where, through visualisation, I take people into their playful selves and then guide them to create an environment in their minds where there are toys and kids' activities for them to get into. Quite often someone will say: 'This is the first time I've realised how little play or how few toys I had in my own childhood. It feels very strange to be playing now; I'm not used to it, but I like it. It feels good'. Participants say much the same thing when I bring out actual toys in the group; as with the visualisation exercise, it can suddenly occur to them that no matter what else, they had missed out on play or enough play or appropriate play.

If people have experienced little or no play in their early years they have often been challenged in playing with and relating to their own children. But though they may be long past childhood themselves, the potential is always there for developing the capacity to play. One of the best things you

One way to access your playful self at home is to get together some drawing paper and coloured crayons. Start drawing with your non-dominant hand (the one you don't use to write) – doodling, making shapes and patterns or specific objects. Just let the pictures form themselves and enjoy your creative output. Don't judge what you are coming out with, just enjoy the childlike feeling of doing. (Why should finger-painting be reserved for children? That's probably even more fun!)

Some other childlike activities you could also try are eating fairy floss, making fairy bread, skipping, bouncing a ball. In my laughter-training workshops we explore some of the games we enjoyed as kids, such as Simon says, hide-and-seek, hopscotch, follow the leader, cowboys. Great fun. Such messing around will probably bring up a host of memories of your childhood: what else you used to play, who you used to play with and where. There's no need to give up the good feelings you enjoyed then. It's all part of the same spectrum.

can do with children is play with them; it's fun and at the same time you'll be helping yourself.

Going too far

Just as there are people who have repressed their playful self there are those whose inner child is overdeveloped! The practical jokers, the people who are constantly seeking attention and the person who does nothing but joke, could possibly be using this mechanism to hide some painful experiences.

Those whose playful self is compulsively outrageous may need to unravel why their behaviour is as it is and what this gained for them as children. Did they go over the top in order to attract attention or were they encouraged by adults who also thought that attention-seeking behaviour was okay? Their task is to understand that it is not always appropriate to give our playful selves absolute free reign. It's how and when we do, that is of value to us: the energy and willingness to be amused and spontaneous are sufficient to keep life pretty interesting.

Enjoying your own humour

When we make full use of our sense of humour we find that we enjoy laughing with others, even people we don't know! Laughter is a great temporary bond. It's impossible to feel hostile towards, or nervous of, someone with whom we can share a genuine laugh.

When we are joined in laughter, we share intimacy. Such moments may be part of our relationship with that person or they may be a fleeting mutuality with strangers. It doesn't matter; they happened and they are valuable to us. Shared laughter brings us closer together; it's a communication that can bridge cultural, age, class, language and sexual barriers and that can leave us feeling good.

Sometimes we find our humour in the company of others. Sometimes we enjoy humour in our own company. Part of the challenge of doing or appreciating something laughter-inducing on our own lies in the way we have been conditioned. Some people grow up connecting laughter with sitting watching a TV program or video or a stage where someone else is deliberately being funny. The canned laughter on TV or the live audience around us seems to give us permission to laugh. Many people are not comfortable laughing when alone, with themselves as both creator and audience. That's a pity.

Creating something funny or frivolous ourselves for our own amusement is just a matter of practice. Initially it may feel rather strange, but then you will realise that being alone – it could be at home, in the car, in the street, in a public place with lots of others – need not be a barrier to having fun.

The concepts in this book are meant to be USED, regularly. Take time out to do them, alone and with others, and to play with the new ideas for having fun which will occur to you from now on. Adapt the suggestions – both my own and those of people from my groups – and make them your own.

You could:

- do five minutes a day of laugh aerobics (including 'Tee hee, Ha ha');
- buy a fun item for your workspace or kitchen;
- keep a record of happenings that make you feel good (see page 8/,,
- arrange to see a comedy on stage or screen;
- hire a funny video;
- meet with a friend with whom you can share some laughs; and
- start collecting cartoons, jokes, sayings, photos (making up speech balloons or writing new captions to them is fun) that appeal to you; display them where they'll remind you to laugh.

Participants in my workshops who do each week's homework claim that their lives and perspectives have changed for the better. They find that the only limit is their imagination and willingness to explore more of those areas of life that yield fun (which is pretty well all of them, when you look at things in a humorous light).

Most of us don't physically need to learn how to laugh; laughing is easy. It's the thinking process that gets in the way, the *notion* of laughing, that can block us.

The first step

Taking the first step is probably the most challenging. It's not a difficult thing to do, but if we believe something is hard then that's what we will experience. It's basically a matter of putting an idea into action, with the task being the link between the two. All it takes is a willingness to alter your perspective about the way you view something.

So examine your attitude and soften it up a bit if you feel you need to. Allow a few new ideas to drift uncensored into your mind, play with them mentally for a while, give them a chance to interact with your existing patterns of behaviour and response. Permit them to guide you to a willingness to try, experiment, give it a go. Be prepared to be silly and absurd; don't censor yourself and don't necessarily conform. Be an independent thinker and laugher.

Because I work with laughter and want to know all about it, I continually stretch my own comfort zones and explore new ways to break through constrictions. This keeps me on my toes and reminds me what it's like for more inhibited people to do challenging things. When I achieve something I thought I couldn't, I feel like I've climbed a mountain, even if it's only a little hill.

This is how I find myself wearing a red nose to the supermarket or a rubber duck's bill while having lunch with a friend, or sporting a (trick) safety pin through my nose. I know it all sounds rather extreme and not something most people would do, but that's not what it's all about. It's about getting past something like a fake nose so you can get past the fear of looking foolish, which is a major reason why people suppress their sense of fun and laughter.

Gibberish and Wiffpiff (see pages 56–60) are terrific 'loosening up' exercises which I use a lot to help people access some new ways of having fun. The aim of Gibberish and Wiffpiff is to engage the brain in a fun and nonsensical activity to alleviate stress and over-seriousness. They allow us to retreat to a childlike state and just fool around with our mouths and our tongue, the way children often do.

People like people who like to laugh. It makes them feel good too. The strange thing is, those who laugh a lot are not necessarily those to whom life has been kindest. They are the folk who accept life's adversities and who use humour to rise above them.

PS: The good thing about being seen as a happy, laughing sort of person is that others are more sympathetic to them when they are occasionally down because they know they are not easily upset.

Laughter and creativity

Although what specifically makes us laugh is different for everyone, there are various triggers that are pretty well common to us all. These are:

- the spontaneous recognition of what is funny;
- our personal source of memory; and
- our own imagination and creativity.

While few would argue with the first two, many people believe they lack the faculties of imagination and creativity. That's untrue: we all have these within us, no matter how underdeveloped or overlaid they may be. When we learn to tap in to our own sources of inspiration, we find we don't have to wait for others or for outside circumstances to provide us with a good laugh. We can do it for ourselves. Like imagination, creativity is also stimulated by laughter – it's circular.

Basically, the skill of being creative – to do with laughter or anything else – lies in taking your knowledge and information and talents, and toying with new ideas and possibilities, letting the mind run free of censorship. Creativity isn't restricted to those normally most connected with creativity: artists, writers, composers, inventors, scientists and the like. We can all be creative – at work, at home, in the garden, in an extracurricular activity, just by making or doing virtually anything.

So if you're looking for new ideas, a fresh approach, avoid telling yourself that there is a right and a wrong way to do something; that you must follow the rules no matter what; that something is not logical; that you are wasting time; that someone like yourself doesn't come up with anything creative.

Sometimes we deliberately seek a creative solution to a problem, other times we suddenly see a creative aspect to something we weren't necessarily looking to change. On occasion a change in routine or expectation is forced upon us, and after lamenting the need to alter our previous focus we discover that what we have come up with is better than the original. A sign of creativity is not to reject a new idea when it comes but to play around with it, finding out how far you can take it.

Play, laughter, activity (which can be as ordinary as going for a walk), and letting your mind freewheel, can stimulate creativity. Humour works to facilitate the flow of ideas and puts you in a mood conducive to ordering and linking unconnected ideas and facts. As we saw in the previous chapter, when we laugh we release hormones that balance the left and right sides of the brain, a boost for the creative process.

We are all far more creative than we give ourselves credit for. If we can create mental monsters – worries, fears, catastrophes that have not yet happened and probably never will but which can be very real to us – we can use the same powers to create thoughts and happenings that we welcome and enjoy. If we have the capacity to wallow in misery, we also have the tools to wallow in joy.

Imagination and visualisation are very close. Imagine (create) positive images for yourself and you'll start to move towards them.

What prevents us from laughing?

If laughing and fun are good for our health and a source of wellbeing, how is it that we don't laugh more often, that many of us even dole out smiles somewhat reluctantly? There are many reasons why we may not help ourselves to the benefits of laughter as frequently as we could. Here are some of the things that we may consciously or unconsciously be saying to ourselves:

- I'm so used to feeling bad; laughing and feeling good are so foreign to me.
- Laughing is noisy and making a noise is undesirable.
- Life is a struggle. What is there to laugh about?
- I shouldn't laugh at a time/place like this.
- People will think I'm crazy if I laugh whenever I feel like it.
- Unless the rest of my life is okay, it's not worth laughing at anything much.
- There has to be a reason to laugh; I can't just create one.
- My laugh is weird. It's better not heard too often.
- My parents/family wouldn't have laughed in particular circumstances and I can't shake off that influence.
- I feel silly if I'm the only person in certain situations who finds something to laugh at.
- Others will reject me if I laugh too much.
- My work is very important to me and I can't see how laughing fits into the workplace.

I'm sure you can add to these examples from your own life. On top of such messages we give ourselves as adults, we can all probably remember as children absorbing negative admonitions about laughter such as: 'Wipe that smile off your face', 'Stop smirking', 'How dare you laugh', and 'Small things amuse small minds'.

Here are some reasons why you may be setting the limitations outlined in the list above. How many can you identify with? Are there any more influences you can think of?

- Childhood messages
- Culture and home environment
- Instilled belief systems
- Taboos
- Peer pressure
- Education system
- Social pressure
- Stress
- Loss and grief
- Fear of looking foolish
- Fear of revealing too much; of having one's values questioned
- Fear of seeming frivolous or inefficient, especially at work
- Religious influences
- Shyness and inhibition
- Fear of losing control
- Unresolved psychological issues.

It's virtually never too late to give yourself permission to laugh more: the oldest person to attend my workshops was eighty-five years old! (More about her on page 60.) Consider these lists, think about what's stopping you and why, and then take some steps to see things differently. One of the best ways of doing this is to start using affirmations.

'Laughaffirmations'

As you may know, affirmations are short, positive messages that we can say over and over to ourselves in order to improve our lives. They are an excellent way to re-program the subconscious, in this instance to enjoy more laughter. If you doubt that such a technique could be effective, just think of the negative messages we tend to give ourselves and which work very effectively to depress and disturb us.

Along the path to becoming someone who laughs often and easily, I recommend you introduce 'laughaffirmations' into your routine so that you consider laughter a healthy and desirable part of life. Say the ones you choose dozens of times a day and you'll start to believe them.

Here are some of the laughaffirmations I have found useful:

- I love to laugh.
- I have a wonderful laugh.
- Laughter heals me.
- When I laugh, the world is a wonderful place.
- Laughing comes easily to me.
- It's fine to laugh.
- Laughter connects me with others.
- I am a humorous person.
- I am a good laugher.
- I can laugh whenever I want to.
- I find it easy to laugh.
- I am a spontaneous person.
- I have a great sense of humour.
- I choose to laugh frequently.
- I am responsible for the humour I perceive.
- There are endless ways I can achieve laughter and create joyful feelings.

You may like to make up your own laughaffirmations to suit your personal situation. Of course, you can also use affirmations to change your attitudes about any other areas of your life that need a push towards positivity.

Many of us grew up thinking that laughing was immature, something that should be controlled and not indulged in as adults in the 'wrong' circumstances. Heaven forbid we should find laughter at work, in church, at funerals and other solemn occasions, at official functions, in public, among strangers and so on! It's easy to see how for some people laughter could be connected in their minds with 'doing the wrong thing'.

3 Laugh aerobics

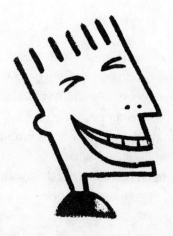

There are three ways I work with others in bringing more laughter into life. All these have contributed to what I call laugh aerobics.

The first is to present myself as a sort of role model. There's nothing more special about me than anyone else, but as a human being on the path of life I have survived a great deal of trauma and pain, and sometimes real hardships.

Before I began the journey to self-awareness and developing my spirituality, I dealt with and surmounted these situations in the best way I could with the tools and understanding I had at the time. Sometimes, as it turned out, that coping strategy was laughter. Sometimes, I felt I could do nothing to help myself. Since I've begun to study and work with laughter, I have drawn more and more on the source of what I teach. I've found that laughter really does work; it has seen me through the tough times and made them easier. (And of course it has enhanced the good times, and often created them.)

A matter of doing

As I have turned around what has been at times a rather difficult life by drawing on the healing and creative power of humour, it's now easy for me to *say* all that I have to say. The challenge comes when it's a matter of *doing*.

The second way I work is to read and research everything I can find on the subject of humour and what it can do. I then discuss these findings in my talks, workshops and seminars, presenting the data as persuasive tools people can use in order to immediately start feeling better. My listeners are left in no doubt that these are not just my own opinions; I let them know that humour and its effects comprise a widespread, legitimate field of study and one that is yielding very positive information.

The medical and associated health-care professions now acknowledge that good health is more than the absence of illness. Not being ill is not necessarily good health. Good health is having a positive response to the world and all that happens to you.

Extending the comfort zone

The third way in which I work is the real fun for me because that's where I witness real change. Through invention, developing concepts, adopting and adapting ideas, and playing and experimenting, I have come up with a range of activities that are laughter-inducing. By introducing participants to all sorts of silly and funny things that get groups going, that gently prise people away from their usual patterns of reacting and behaving, I lead them to have a good time – even in the midst of strangers (as they often are, at least when they start out).

Some of the things we get up to are, quite frankly, pretty ridiculous nonsense, but it's amazing how they work. As I have explained, I don't expect others to perform such antics, but there is value in their seeing me as a middle-aged woman allowing herself to be silly and not embarrassed.

One way you can start broadening your comfort zone is at home; you'll probably be surprised to find how you've been fencing yourself in. There's no one to see you, so let yourself go: wear a silly hat, sing loudly, laugh out loud, kiss your hands and arms (see page 70), tune in to a TV or radio program that amuses you. It will put you in the mood to extend the feelings of wellbeing and confidence to the world outside.

You can do all the following laugh aerobics at home, at work or in a group. They are designed to be done not once but often, so that you get used to laughing with them and are prepared for other laughs. It is a matter of developing the humour habit.

Gibberish

Talking gibberish is particularly effective in getting people laughing and interacting. When I outline the idea to my students they often claim that they won't be able to do it, that they'd feel ridiculous, and so on. The only skill that's required is a willingness to try. As soon as people do, they and others find it a lot of fun.

If you tell yourself that you can't talk gibberish – that you're too serious, you're not a laugher – imagine what else you're telling yourself you can't do. Catch yourself in the thinking process and you'll find you're probably saying 'I won't' rather than 'I can't'.

Gibberish is most effective when you have an idea of what you are talking about, rather than just making up words or sounds. Decide what you want to say – it can be anything at all – and use arm, hand and facial gestures to go with it. Two people having an animated conversation in gibberish is a hoot for all concerned. You can also talk gibberish out loud to yourself or even sing it.

In gibberish you use sounds and syllables only; this can include animal sounds such as 'miaow-miaow' and 'woof woof', and meaningless sounds such as 'la la', 'huh?' and so on. Lots of expression brings this 'language' to life. So start talking nonsense (the way a foreign language can sound) by connecting sounds, vowels, consonants and syllables in an unstructured way.

For example, you could make up words such as 'cookoo', 'lamiaw', 'fuli', 'mucky lanamacar', 'yuiki ooki', 'yum yum', 'oo oo', 'frista'. These you could supplement with guttural sounds and noises from your throat like 'ee', 'errr', 'ahrhhh' and then you could repeat them in conjunction with a series of gestures and dramatic punctuation as if you really wished to communicate. The experience of being expressive and animated with your face, hands and body is excellent for conditioning you to use all of your being in a fun way.

Some people (particularly some children) are terrific gibberishers and can rattle off a whole dialogue as if it means something. I'm quite good at it too, and often have a complete and nonsensical conversation with group participants, much to the amusement of others. See how spontaneous and creative *you* can be and enjoy the laughter that will bubble up in yourself and in others. You'll quickly lose your self-consciousness once you get into the swing of it. The main thing is, if it feels fun, keep doing it.

Victor Borge, the Danish pianist humourist, is a master of phonetic punctuation. He makes different sounds for full stops, commas, dashes, question marks and inverted commas, so that a simple dialogue reading can be hilarious.

Years ago (when I used to go and see his stage shows), I'd copy his phonetic punctuations in reading bedtime stories to my friends' children. They loved it so much they didn't want the stories to end. I virtually had to be rescued by their parents.

What I said went something like this: 'Click click (a clicking sound coming from the back of the teeth), what are you doing little red riding hood niyeh prt click click going to see my grandma and I'm taking a food basket click click'. My young listeners used to roar with joy and laughter at this nonsense.

I find that some people feel that having fun is difficult, something they'd like to do if they could except that often it's too hard. Finding fun for them is like extracting teeth. They come up with all sorts of explanations for the barriers they have erected: 'I don't have time', 'I don't want to look silly', 'Fun is for kids', 'I haven't had fun for years and I don't know how to get into it' or saddest of all, 'I don't know what you mean'. They leave fun to chance and when it temporarily deserts them they permanently turn their backs on it.

Wiffpiff

Wiffpiff is a bit different. It usually has people in workshops breaking into laughter before they even try it. I derived the word Wiffpiff from the word 'lisping' and lisping is what this is.

(Incidentally, in my workshops I've never had anyone with a speech impediment indicate that hearing the rest of us deliberately speaking in Wiffpiff offended them at all. The opposite is true, in fact. One woman's comment is typical. Although she had a very pronounced lisp she entered into Wiffpiff with gusto, saying afterwards that she felt she was easily understood and that for the first time in her life she had fun sharing her way of speaking.)

Here's how to speak in Wiffpiff: curl your tongue downward and press it against your lower teeth so that the curled tongue takes up as much space in your mouth as possible. This will leave you with little room for clarity of speech. Then try to speak as you usually do! The result is very funny.

When I'm demonstrating this potential for fun in a group I usually ask participants to say in Wiffpiff what they had for breakfast. 'Coffee and totht', they reply. 'Exth and bakern.' Sounds silly, and it is, but it's also hilarious and gets the most straightlaced people going. They revert to a childlike state: you can see the little kid in them; their faces, even their bodies, change.

Sometimes in my classes I set as homework a written piece of Wiffpiff. It's something you can do too and I guarantee you'll end up chuckling. Below is the contribution of James, a student of mine. James came to the workshops to help heal the hurt of his separation from his wife and children. Sometimes he was very sad, other times he let himself enter into the fun and nonsense in a wholehearted manner. It was wonderful to see as the weeks went by his playful self emerging and cheering him up at a difficult time. This is what he wrote:

> Laffink ith thudth a walleeth. It ith a thotahally atteptbool way of wetting go of eveweyday tenthon and thtweth. But laffink dothend ddutht happen, you haff to giff yourthelff permithon to waff. De pawent in you hath to thtop dominating and wet the thild out to pway. Thith can be confwuntin becoorth the thild dothent wear any mathkths, ethept thorow (Zorro) and Batman mathkths and they're weal fun. Becoorth you can be whoever you want and thange ath muth ath you wike and haff fun and laff.

Get in touth with your ability to laff and you will have more fun in yure life. Yeth, there will thtill be pain and thadneth but you will be hedda eqwipt to deal with all athpeth of your life if you allow yourthelf to laff.

By Gweg.

P.Eth. My toungue is thore from wyting.

I particularly recall a charming eighty-five-year-old woman who came along to a one-day seminar I held (she is the oldest workshop participant I've had, although there have been plenty in their sixties and seventies). She told us she had not laughed much for a number of years, in fact not since her husband had died. Even when she watched something funny on television, she said that she felt silly and guilty sitting there on her own and laughing out loud.

As the day proceeded she began to do the funny and silly things we got into, and started to enjoy herself. By the time we came to Wiffpiff, she was able to enter into it wholeheartedly. She laughed so much talking in Wiffpiff that her false teeth fell out. She had a second try, and they fell out again! She laughed uproariously.

It was wonderful to witness the change and to hear her say that she now realised that any reason to laugh is good and that she would allow herself to do far more of it in future.

Singing funly

Along with the gift of laughter, nature was also generous in giving us all natural singing voices. For good reason, because singing – no matter how badly – is a freeing, happy, intensely personal experience. Like laughing, it is a great way to express ourselves, to push back the boundaries and to have fun.

Yet because some of us may not have voices that are harmonious or trained or whatever, is no reason not to use them. Probably quite a number of us sang when we were younger, perhaps in a choir or just for fun. As we get older, we tend to judge our voices and stop creating the harmony we used to enjoy. (Sadly, probably the only time many adults sing is half-heartedly pretending to participate in the national anthem or in group singing such as Christmas carols.)

Again, it's just a matter of giving yourself permission to do anything you like that feels good and that doesn't harm others (the only thing you can hurt here is the ears). If you're really self-conscious about your voice, sing only when alone – in the shower, in the car, while walking.

What initially showed me the value of singing badly was when a very sad man, whom I'll call Fred, came to one of my workshops. He had recently learned of a serious illness. Fred said he would have loved to be able to sing away his blues but he felt he couldn't because he sang so badly.

I tried to reassure him that it didn't matter what he sounded like but he was unconvinced. So I had the idea to ask the members of the class to stand together with Fred and sing 'Jingle Bells'. I asked them to assume a singer's stance for the event.

'Stand up very straight', I said. 'Put your shoulders back and clasp your hands together at chest level, just like opera singers do when they are about to burst into an aria. Wiggle a bit to get into position, pucker up the lips, make some sounds – such as "mimimimi", as if you are about to deliver something tuneful – and launch into it.' I instructed them to deliberately sing loudly, off-key, out of tune, out of time and as badly as they could screech.

Off we went, sounding rather like a pack of cats on heat, a cacophony of squeaking and crackling and distortion . . . But was it FUN! Everyone started laughing and didn't want to stop, so we sang some more. When we finally finished we all felt great, happy, relaxed and stimulated.

Fred himself said he felt liberated. I gave him singing badly as his homework and he now felt he could carry it out. The next meeting he came along looking happier, reporting that the week had been the best he'd had for a long time and that he had kept up his task, particularly in the car. (I like to sing in the car too and sometimes I forget the words so I sing in gibberish.)

Have you ever hummed (or sung) a tune as you were walking down the street, then looked around to see if anyone was around to hear you? Don't stop yourself if you feel like bursting into song; it's a wonderful way to enjoy yourself, and blow what anyone thinks. (They'll probably envy your spontaneity.)

I don't agree with the messages we were given as children when, through persuasion, punishment, disencouragement and disincentive, we were led to believe that if we couldn't do something properly or well, it wasn't worth bothering with.

Now that you're an adult, you can sing how you like – loudly, off-key, out of tune, out of time, well or badly. Be as creative as you like with the words (make up your own lyrics, too) and the music; the only person you need to consider is yourself. (A tip: my students have found that a particularly good song to have fun with is the Bee Gees' 'Stayin' Alive', with its falsetto sections.)

Laughter line

This is a useful exercise for helping you tune in to your feelings concerning your life at the moment.

Picture a line several metres long on the floor. One end represents 'Lots of laughter', the other 'Nothing to laugh about'. See the middle of the line as being a neutral 'Okay', place. Walk along the line, stopping at the point that best represents you and your life at the moment. Get in touch with that feeling.

If you've indicated 'Lots of laughter', enjoy where you're at, knowing that you're in good emotional shape. If you've chosen the other end of the line, make a conscious decision to walk towards 'Lots of laughter'. Even a few small steps towards the middle marks a physical shift towards feeling better. Sometimes we can use our bodies to take us where our minds need to go.

Temper tantrums

Temper tantrums receive bad press. Nobody likes them in children or adults; they are unwelcome to the observer and painful to the tantrum-thrower.

Yet there is something to be said for temper tantrums. Carried out with a particular focus – releasing stress or excising uncomfortable memories or dealing with anger towards someone or something – they can be very useful for getting rid of negative energy that can build up and cause all sorts of problems if not healthily discharged.

As part of your journey towards greater enjoyment of life, you may choose to have a planned tantrum to clear yourself of these suppressions. Find a quiet and private place where you can make noise and move around as you need. Really get into who or what is bothering you and let yourself get incredibly angry. Yell, stamp, thrash about, roll on the floor, if you like. Act like a thwarted two- or three-year-old for several minutes until you feel cleansed and ready to calm down. You may experience a range of feelings before this happens and it is quite likely you will want to cry at some point. Don't hold yourself back in any way – get it all out.

Repeat this exercise as often as necessary. Participants in my workshops who carry out these planned tantrums at home report that they actually come to regard them as fun as well as valuable. Some people even report that they share a tantrum with a friend.

The sounds of your body

This is another good exercise for getting in touch with your body and yourself. It will help you identify what stress you are carrying in your body and to start to release it. Do it on your own or in a group situation.

Stand straight, eyes closed. Take a few deep breaths and visualise your body. Bring your mind to your toes, breathe in and on the 'out' breath let sounds emerge from your mouth – any sounds at all. Repeat this process for your knees, genitals, navel, chest, shoulders, neck, face, scalp and any other places that need to express themselves.

Taking your body for a walk

This is a group or individual exercise that also will help you get in touch with your body and have fun with it. It makes you aware of the way your body and mind work, separately and together, and how you can influence them through your activities. Greater awareness of how and why you move and act will make you more aware of yourself and the fact that we take so much for granted.

Stroll briskly around the room or any other designated area. Talk aloud to your body as you go along. Tell your feet which way to go; compliment them on how well they are doing and express how much you appreciate their taking you wherever you want to go. Have a similar chat with your legs. Praise your arms for the part they play and your eyes for showing you the way. You can end up by thanking your voice for being there to comment on your walk.

Laughter symphony

This exercise uses various laughter syllables to get a large or small (minimum of three) group loosened up and laughing.

Divide the group into three equal parts. One sub-group will sing 'Hee hee hee' in high voices (soprano), another will sing 'Ha ha ha' in middling voices (mezzo), and the last group will sing 'Ho ho ho' in low voices (baritone).

Choose a suitable tune and pick an orchestra leader. His or her job is to conduct the various groups as they make their designated sounds to the music (instead of words). The leader can decide whether to bring the groups in at the same time or at different times. However it is done a joyful cacophony is guaranteed to be the outcome.

The good feelings generated can then be harnessed into a laughter competition. Each of the three groups does a group laugh. The funniest (for others) and most contagious wins.

Bringing down the 'Ha ha' energy

This activity can be done in a group or by yourself, perhaps following your morning laugh aerobics exercises.

Stand straight with your legs comfortably apart and take some deep, slow breaths. Close your eyes if you feel a bit uncomfortable in a group. (You may find doing this will help you concentrate.)

Imagine that a few inches above your head is a huge, endless amount of feel-good energy. Now slowly lift your arms up towards it, up, up, stretch, it's almost within reach, you can get it. Ah, you've got a grasp on it. Good. Now pull it down all over you, feel it covering and enveloping you and going in through your pores, reaching to your very centre. Experience it doing you good; know that it will stay with you.

Tell yourself this store of feel-good energy will keep you buoyed and cheerful all day and will help you to tap in to fun and laughter more easily. It's also there to call on if specific situations start to get you down.

Tarzan

Research has shown that when we laugh we cause the thymus gland (located in the upper chest) to produce endorphins, the hormones that give us a feeling of wellbeing.

Tarzan knew something when he dashed about thumping his chest and making his unique call (very like the sounds I recommend to get you into laughing mode). So borrow his idea and thump your thymus with both hands and with great relish and let out a great loud 'Ah aha hahaaaaaa'!

Another exercise that gets the thymus going is to pretend you are conducting an orchestra. (Research into the health and longevity of many conductors indicates that thymus stimulation plays a large role in this.) Put on some music (*Bolero* or a selection from *Aida* are ideal, as is anything with a strong and regular beat) and imagine you are a famous conductor in front of an orchestra. Really bend your body and arms and head to the music and to bring in the different instruments. When I conduct, I'm so absorbed I almost touch the floor! The feeling afterwards is terrific – guaranteed to get rid of the most negative thoughts and to energise and uplift.

Feeling good about yourself

In the pursuit of laughter, a major component (I've come to realise) is self-esteem. When we feel good about ourselves and who we are and are at ease with ourselves, laughter can come easily. And when we have come to terms with the sounds of our laughter, developing our own brand of humour becomes important to us.

Developing self-esteem is as much a journey as laughter is. At the core of it is the belief that 'I am a worthwhile person'. No matter who you are or what you do or where you come from, you are always a worthwhile person; a wonderful, unique and remarkable human being. Simply because you are on the planet at this time makes you worthwhile. What's happened to you, where you've been, what you've done, what you've learnt, what you've become, and the opportunities, challenges and processes by which your life has unfolded to date, have made you what you are – and this is always worthwhile.

Sometimes to really understand this and to absorb it we need the assistance of some therapy, a good friend or some other way of connecting with ourselves. For me, this path has been realising that there is a vast universal energy that I tap in to and am part of. A higher spirit connects me with joy and peace. Each of us pursues and finds peace and joy in our own way. I do encourage you to develop ways and means of appreciating yourself JUST AS YOU ARE.

Value about yourself all that is good and wonderful. Part of this will be your humour. When we feel relaxed and happy with ourselves we are more likely to engage in light-hearted activities that go to make us feel even better.

The following simple and accessible exercises will enhance your appreciation of yourself and show you how to make the most of everything (no matter how small) that is good and that makes you feel good. I suggest that you don't censor yourself but that you experience just what these exercises can do for you!

Standing ovation

You deserve some appreciation! You generally do such a good job that you are due a great big pat on the back from your family, your work colleagues, your friends and any others around you.

The chances are that you won't get it unless you let them know that you would like one. So do it! In fact, go further and ask for a standing ovation; stand up on a chair to receive it. Everyone applauds you, stands and cheers wildly and yells 'Encore, encore!'

This exercise is also to do with self-appreciation. You don't need a reason to ask for it. It doesn't need to be a pat on the back for doing or being something. It's just for being. A standing ovation is an excellent opportunity for those around you to give unconditionally.

This exercise teaches you to ask for what you want, to recognise that you are worthy of expressed approval and to enjoy it when it comes. You don't have to have done anything specific to ask for a standing ovation: you merely have to feel you'd like one. Perhaps you could organise a standing ovation for someone else and help raise their self-esteem. It's a fabulous feeling both to receive and to give a standing ovation.

Bring the standing ovation into the workplace – in staff-rooms, boardrooms and offices. The feedback I have received from this has been quite amazing. It's a good way for colleagues to give and receive appreciation.

Kiss your hands

Your hands are an accessible part of you and therefore easy to concentrate on.

First, look at your hands. Examine them as though this is the very first time you have seen hands. Look at their shape, colour, texture and the features that make them yours – dimples, knobs, bumps, veins, cuts, lines, nails, jewellery.

Think of all that your hands do for you in the course of a day. They wash you, dress you, feed you (and others), care for your house and body, help you earn a living, write, stroke, pat, scratch, wave and even speak for you.

Let yourself realise how lucky you are to have these remarkable hands. Let yourself know how much you love them by kissing them. Start with the fingertips and work your way around the palms and the backs, up to the wrists. If you really get into it, you can go up your arm as well. Enjoy the appreciation you are giving your precious hands and the fun way you are going about it.

By kissing your hands, you are connecting with loving yourself. Do this exercise as often as you like, whenever you like, simply as a reminder that the same appreciation is due to the rest of your body, your being. Sneaking a little smooch to your fingers when someone is giving you a hard time (excellent for the workplace) is a great way to switch on your good feelings about yourself.

Inner body laugh visualisation

In the first chapter we looked at how and why laughing is so good for the body. In order to keep our insides toned by the effect of laughter I've developed this inner body laugh visualisation, also known as laughing kinaesthetically.

Just as sportspeople, musicians, people doing exams and performers sometimes rehearse their performances in their minds, we too can visualise ourselves laughing. It sets us up for the real thing. More than that, it really gives the body a work-out as, strangely, the benefits are there even though you haven't gone through the physical process.

I believe the visualisation is an important process because it enables the mind to guide the body's health and healing and confers the ability to see oneself laughing all through our being. Imagine that by seeing in your mind various parts

This is a useful exercise for a group to do, aimed particularly at those who haven't laughed properly for a long time or who are inhibited about laughing.

Stand holding the belly with both palms, pulling the shoulders back and rocking backwards and forwards, letting out a lot of 'Hahahaha' sounds. It's important at this point to make quite a lot of noise as some people laugh silently (having been discouraged from laughing noisily when young). A good way for them to find their voice is in a group of people all letting go with a lot of happy sounds.

of the body laughing you are teaching your very cells to have a better perception of laughter and its amazing properties. This visualisation is also very good for the serious-minded because it internalises the whole process of laughter.

The activity is especially useful for those who are bed- or chair-bound or who have an injury or disability. I have introduced it to good effect to the elderly, to people with multiple sclerosis and cancer, to children, to company executives. It's a personal and private laughter time, whether you do it in a group or by yourself.

Start by finding a comfortable place to sit (or lie). Make yourself really comfortable, close your eyes and, if you are sitting, put your feet flat on the ground and your hands in your lap.

Let your breath rise and fall, in and out. Notice your breath going in and out of your nose; be conscious of this for several breaths and feel yourself relaxing and sinking into your seat.

Next, imagine a spot about four fingers' width down from your navel. Visualise this spot as deep inside you and orange in colour like the fruit. Focus on the colour and size of this spot, and in your mind make it bigger and fluid-like until it becomes a warm orange-coloured tide that flows throughout your whole body.

Feel this happy liquid running through every cell and corpuscle, filling you with joy and the desire to laugh. Keep this up until you have a very clear picture in your mind of what your insides now look like.

Then picture yourself wearing a big smile and laughing heartily. SEE IT! See your mouth in a happy shape, your eyes crinkled with laughter, the top of your nose wrinkled in laughter, your cheeks round and cherubic as you really get into it. Hear the happy sound you are making. Feel this laugh taking hold of your shoulders and chest, your diaphragm going up and down with mirth, your whole body down to your legs and feet responding to the mirth. See you clutching yourself in this cosmic chuckle! You may find that your body actually does start to shake and move in accordance with what your mind is conjuring up.

Continue to breathe deeply as you imagine laughter and joy taking you over.

Keep the laughter going and journey further into yourself. What we are doing now is sending the healing energy of laughter to specific organs and enjoying the thought of all those helpful endorphins doing their bit to put you in good shape.

Imagine the mirth affecting your lungs and your heart, giving them a good work-out; picture the blood vessels and liver going in and out in time with the spasms. See your stomach having a good time; it will help your digestion. Feel the effect on your muscles, relaxing and strengthening them. Focus on any particular parts of the body that have been giving you trouble, not working well, and imagine them having a good time and functioning perfectly. Orchestrate your whole being as if you were conducting a great symphony.

But we're not finished yet. Let's go deeper now. See your skeleton, your brain, your bones, your cells all joining in. You are full of laughter. See if you can deepen it yet further, feel more of it. Stay in this wonderful place and savour how great you feel, breathing in and out, deeply and slowly.

When you are ready, gradually bring your mind back to the present and open your eyes by degrees. You should be feeling on top of the world and full of laughter, as indeed you are full of laughter. Move on to your next activity or just continue to bask in the afterglow.

You can do this meditation any time you like, as often as you like. If you don't always have time for the whole body to be involved just visualise the major parts and effects. It is important that you see what is happening when you laugh heartily, particularly if you have got out of the habit of laughing or are self-conscious about the way you look or sound when you laugh. If you are doing the exercise on your own, you may like to read it first onto tape and let the tape guide you through.

I have found in my workshops that this inner body laugh calls forth a range of responses, each person enjoying the effect on a different imagined part of the body. Nearly everyone finds the practice very beneficial (though inevitably from time to time someone reports that 'nothing happened', which indicates the need to keep practising letting laughter take them over). Overwhelmingly, participants find it leaves them deeply exercised and content – some even fall asleep!

Daily laughter activities

Here are some suggestions for laughter activities you can do every day:

- Start the day with some laugh aerobics, as outlined in this chapter.
- Decide to have a great day.

'I can't do this – what will THEY think of ME?'
'I couldn't behave like that in front of THEM.'

In our own minds and bodies we are all ME and I. THEM and THEY are everybody else – partners, parents, children, workmates, friends, acquaintances, people in shops and in the streets, strangers.

Each THEM and THEY sees themselves as a ME. To others you and I are part of the THEY and THEM who cause all that worry about what they think. Wouldn't it be nice if one of THEM could worry about what the others think of ME and then we could do and be anything we like? We could be silly, have fun, play and laugh and THEY would be worrying about it while ME enjoys itself. What a pity we do it the other way around.

It's important to put THEM, THEY and ME in proper perspective.

- Tell yourself that you are wonderful ten times under the shower.
- Bring to mind one funny incident or anecdote per day.
- Go to work with the expectation of enjoying your work or your activities and the people you come into contact with.
- Have at least one fun or fluffy item in your workspace.
- Genuinely praise others.
- Visualise yourself as a light-hearted person, laughing.

- Develop some self-esteem 'quickies', for example, every day appreciate a different part of yourself; or recall the last time you received praise and savour that time again; or make sure that when you do something well you say to yourself, 'That was excellent (name), thank you'.

4 Letting more laughs into life

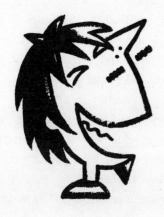

An important component of my work is helping people gain a better insight into their feelings and focusing on how and why they may have unconsciously blocked laughter and that connected reaction, crying. We follow on here from the second chapter, where we considered how earlier restrictions and self-messages had an impact on expressing feelings.

People often tell me what a relief it is to at last identify their state of mind and their attitudes. Thinking about laughter in their lives – and in their childhood – often helps them to understand a great deal about themselves. They've come along to the group because they want to change and now they have some background information to give them perspective. They are ready to learn how to seek out and create opportunities for increasing the amount of fun and laughter in their lives, which in turn can frequently clear other blockages.

Specific blocks to laughter

The following are the type of questions we ask ourselves in workshops about our feelings and the expression of them. Some relate directly to laughter and fun, others to the emotions that are closely allied. Take time to consider them.

- Was there much laughter in my family as a child?
- What were some of the messages I received in childhood about laughter? What do I as an adult believe about laughter?
- Do I think it's okay to laugh when I'm depressed or worried?
- When something sad happens, do I cry?
- What are the things that make me angry? How do I show anger?
- Does laughter come easily to me?
- What sort of things do I find funny? What do I enjoy?
- If someone else is laughing and I don't see the point, how do I feel? What do I do?
- What do I feel about my life right now?
- What are my challenges?
- How can I improve my sense of humour?

There are also other blocks to laughter which you may be grappling with. These could include grief and loss, shyness or even boredom. You can read about these in Chapter 3.

Laughter and stress relief

If you're like the majority of people I meet, it's very likely that you will identify stress in various forms as the reason you don't have more fun or laugh more often.

When circumstances are really against them, even those with a lively sense of humour can find it dampened. Prolonged stress can seem to overwhelm the lighter side of life; we have probably all known times when a sense of joy has seemingly vanished. Understanding what laughter can do for us, even or especially when things are not at their best, is an excellent reason for seeking out and cultivating that release.

It is likely that all of us have encountered difficult personal circumstances at times and found them stress-inducing. Such problems could include financial difficulties; job threat or loss; illness or the death of a loved one; guilt; fear; uncertainty; change; personal ill health; separation or divorce; unsatisfactory living conditions; and so on.

But stress is highly individual too: what stresses me out may not be much of a problem for you and vice versa. When we discuss personal stresses in the laughter-training workshops, people come up with a range of factors that are as varied as they are.

The following are typical of those I've heard:

- Being overweight
- Losing a pet
- Moving house
- Coping with disability
- Loneliness or isolation
- Not having the right clothes for the occasion
- Feeling unattractive
- Too much work or not enough
- Unresolved psychological problems
- Being robbed
- Being a poor cook or housekeeper

- Feeling unloved
- Not being a clever conversationalist
- Not coping with studies
- Being 'stuck' creatively.

Some of these may strike a chord or you may be able to add stresses of your own.

I can't tell you what to laugh about because we are all different and we all lead different lives, but I suggest you be constantly on the lookout for what appeals to you. Observe the way people walk and move, how they dress and look, what they say and what they don't say. Some giggles I have enjoyed in the daily round are: a road sign saying 'Curve', which in one of the languages I speak (Yiddish) means 'prostitute'; a sign at the airport saying 'Revolting doorway'; a young man with bright green hair who caught me looking at him, open-mouthed, and we shared a laugh together.

A great stress-buster

The bottom line is that we all have things in our lives, big and small, that we are grappling with and which are likely to cause stress. As one stressful situation resolves, you can be sure that in due course another will come along. This is part of being human; we can't really escape it. What we can do is develop a humour-armour against feeling that it's all too hard to cope with.

Whatever the source of your particular stress(es), one of the greatest stress-busters around is a good laugh and developing your sense of humour. You'll find that the worry and concern doesn't feel half so bad – even momentarily – if you can find something to laugh at. (Any sort of a laugh is a bonus; best of all is the kind where you shake and bend with it and get an ache in the ribs and tears come to your eyes. Feel it doing you good!)

Everyone starts the journey to laughter from a different point. If you're living with a lot of emotional pain you may wonder how you move from identifying totally with your problems to recognising that there is also a good side to life and allying yourself with it. The answer is to take it slowly, to make small steps, to congratulate yourself each time you let go of a long-time habit or way of thinking. Your desire and capacity to laugh are there all right; the challenge is to learn how to let them come to the surface.

It may be that you can find something in the stressful situation itself to laugh and joke about. It may be that what makes you laugh is quite outside this sphere. The important thing is to make sure you do it, even when you feel least like it.

A worksheet I use in my workshops to help people who feel stuck in a stress situation could also help: first, choose five situations that you are concerned or stressed about. Then take the same five situations and create the worst-case scenarios for them (you'll realise how unlikely these are to occur). And finally, create fun solutions for each of the five situations. They can be things you could really put into motion or things that will make you laugh through their absurdity. Either way, you'll probably no longer be feeling trapped.

It's not hard to believe that in a difficult situation humour can be the best form of temporary stress release. In an interesting piece of research carried out by Cornell University in New York, people who watched a short, funny film and who then tackled some puzzling problems came up with more creative solutions than those who had watched a sober film or who had exercised. In other studies by the same researcher, it was found that after watching comedy films or being involved in an amusing situation, people thought more clearly and were better able to make more informed decisions.

'Off' days

Even in an 'ordinary' life there are ups and downs, good and 'off' days. It's never smooth sailing all the time, for anyone. The scenario that Charlie Brown once described: 'Some days, all the bad days attack me at once' is pretty familiar to me. This is the time to put some of my laughter ideas into action, and I promise they'll help get you out of the doldrums.

At times it's worse than this and we really fall back into the misery pit. Remember it's normal and human to experience all our feelings, to cry or to feel sorry for ourselves on occasion, to resent that too many bad things are happening, to complain that no one cares, to think it's all too difficult.

These suggestions will enable you to get out of a sad or negative mood and move on to creating a better one.

- Project yourself in time, adding a good outcome to a negative situation.
- If you do decide to be miserable, then blow it all out of proportion and enjoy the effect! Be aware of what you are doing and exaggerate the awfulness of it all. Fantasise your situation until it's so bad it becomes totally ludicrous, like a soap opera. The more ridiculous the scenario, the funnier it will become; now you have a marvellous, self-created opportunity to laugh about circumstances that seem overwhelming.

Once (a long time ago), I used to keep emotional diaries. Into them I poured out all the pain, agony and grievances of my life: the diaries served as an observation of myself. When I looked at them later, sometimes years later, I realised what a lot of self-inflicted torture I had put myself through. Although what had happened to me was real, the way I experienced it was the result of my totally wallowing in misery. Now I see how funny some of my agonising was.

I don't mean that we should trivialise our deepest feelings; it's good to be in touch with them and to bring them into the open. Yet I think we can sometimes 'look back in laughter' at what we felt so deeply, often (especially) when we are adolescents or young adults.

These days I'm not sure about the value of keeping an emotional diary; it puts the focus too much on things that hurt. I'd rather deal with them in the present and move on. That's why I've developed what I call the Feel-good Savings Account (explained on pages 86–88). This technique dwells on recording and recalling the positives rather than the negatives of life.

It's important to tune in to your own coping mechanisms when things don't work out the way you'd like them to. Do what you can to climb out of the paralysing inactivity of worry and concerns when life offers you some harsh lessons and painful situations. Measures that help include: being spontaneous; having fun; relaxing; meditating; being aware of what you enjoy about your work, colleagues, friends, family, your environment; and getting a kick out of the things you love.

Despite all the painful things that can occur to us individually and in the world, it is vital to our mental, emotional and physical health that whatever happens we maintain what is important – our interests, our work, our friendships and relationships, and our laughter. They all need nurturing and valuing, even when – especially when – aspects of our lives are not terrific.

I'm sure we've all had the experience of being really upset, perhaps even having a cry, and then something funny occurs or is thought of. Often we fight that impulse to laugh because we're busy being miserable. Be amused for the moment, even if you go back to the blues afterward. Humour is never a wasted emotion.

We will move on (or move back) to our quest to find or make laughter and enjoyment.

In order to be able to see the humour in a situation, especially an upsetting or stressful one, it is usually necessary to step back. It is then that the absurdities emerge. This is a bit different from the process of being able to make a funny story out of a disastrous holiday, for instance. That takes time. Finding humour in a situation in order to lessen stress immediately calls for being able to laugh at things while they are occurring or just after.

One of my favourite recommendations for doing this is to imagine how your favourite cartoon character or comedian would react in similar circumstances. You could even pretend you're the star of a TV comedy and that the frustrating situation is part of the plot you have to make fun out of.

If all else fails, when something bad happens call to mind the old Jewish saying: 'This too shall pass'. It reminds us that we're not stuck there forever.

Humour as a survival mechanism

Even in the midst of the greatest difficulties, many people (like the psychiatrist and Holocaust survivor Victor Frankl who wrote the inspiring *Man's Search for Meaning*) have been able to draw on a sense of humour to keep them going. It has acted as a weapon, an inner resistance; something that couldn't be taken away. The stories of oppressed people who have survived with their humour intact show us that there can be joys and pleasures in virtually anything that happens to us, and indeed *despite* what happens to us.

I have read many accounts of the power of humour to keep people sane in dreadful circumstances. One recent study I came across reported that among Israeli children billeted in unsettled border areas, the lowest rate of psychological problems occurred where they were living with people who demonstrated a sense of humour.

Another piece of research carried out extensive observations of people under intense and prolonged stress. They ranged from children with terminal illnesses to political hostages to overworked executives. It was found that those who withstood the pressures shared three factors: they actively cared about others; they had the capacity to see events from a humorous perspective which enabled them to gain a sense of control and maintain a sense of joy; and they drew support from friends and the community.

The Feel-good Savings Account

In the course of my developing new material, I created the Feel-good Savings Account. It is a useful way of keeping track of the good things in our lives, from the smallest incidents to the major events. It's so easy to overlook or forget the good things that do happen; recording them means they can keep on giving you pleasure.

I'll describe how I keep my account; you may wish to adapt the idea. The important thing is that you keep tabs on all the nice things that happen to you, which probably add up to quite a few every day when you start tuning in to them.

I suggest you buy a small notebook, maybe one that reminds you of a regular bank savings account book. Keep it by the side of your bed, and once a week make entries in it of that week's joys, no matter how minor, before they are gone and forgotten.

My notebook is divided into three columns: the left-hand column is for the date; the middle column (the widest) contains a few words about an event or situation; and the right-hand column attributes a number of points to each entry. The points, on a scale of one to one hundred, indicate

My Feel-good Savings Account

Date	Event or situation	Emotional value (from 1 to 100)
8/3/95	Had lunch with Naomi	80
24/5/95	Received a letter from my brother in France	90
26/6/95	Bought a great new outfit	76
28/6/95	Forgave Mum for everything and at the same time noticed a magnificent rainbow in the sky	100
30/8/95	Finally found a great hairdresser – excellent haircut	85
27/11/95	I lost seven kilos in five weeks	89
12/12/95	Results on leg X-ray not as bad as I had imagined	95

the emotional value you give to the feel-good happening. It is important to focus on this column: how much an event or situation *feels* good really helps us focus on our feelings. You will be surprised how much the happy things meant to you at the time, and how many there are.

When life isn't so wonderful, and even small joys fail to materialise (or more likely you're failing to register them – easy to do if you're feeling down), you have only to look back over your 'deposits' to remind yourself how rich you are. Human nature being what it is, we tend to put to the back of our minds the joy we have recently experienced when we are feeling stressed or miserable.

When something definitely bad does happen to you (as opposed to just being 'blue') the account will also serve to focus your mind on the credits rather than the deficits. Find an entry that particularly appeals to you and deliberately dwell on that instead. Your mind cannot concentrate on two things at once, so fill it with positive feelings rather than hurt, unhappy or negative ones.

It's useful not only to write in your week's quotient of fun on, say, a Sunday night, but at the same time to review the week. You'll be able to see whether you have a balance of work and play, seriousness and humour, duty and fun. If not, plan some good – even silly or outrageous – things for the following week.

A matter of attitude

Like choosing to laugh, we can choose to be positive, to have a good attitude. A simple way of looking at attitude is to understand that we can respond to difficult situations in

When we laugh at someone doing something unexpected and unintentional, such as slipping on a banana skin or similar, our response is a spontaneous reaction made up of various elements. One is probably 'Thank goodness this has not happened to me', and another is the amusement of seeing arms and legs going in all directions and the person falling down in a heap. Such an incident is full of tension, not only for the person involved but for onlookers, and we laugh to relieve that tension. Our appreciation of the humour is increased where the victim can laugh at themselves too.

a number of ways. We can say 'This is hard' or we can say 'This is a challenge, let's see if I can learn something here'.

Being able to see the humour in something – from the things that happen to us or others, to nonsense, jokes, anecdotes, cartoons, funny films and books or whatever else turns us on – is largely a matter of attitude as well as taste.

We are so used to whingeing, to what Robert Holden (see pages 117–18) calls 'not-so-baditis'. On top of that, many people lack a positive, joyous attitude even when nothing much is wrong in their lives. It's my belief that children should be taught in primary school that positive emotions are therapeutic, fostering good health, boosting the immune system and hastening recovery from illness.

Since attitude is fundamentally important to determining the way we view ourselves and others, how we approach our health and wellbeing, the things that motivate us and our moods and responses, it may sound like something that is fixed, like the colour of our eyes, and that it can never change. The good news about attitude is that you can change it. Make a decision that fun and laughter and feeling good are going to be part of your daily world. Have the courage and the commitment to do everything you can to make it so.

Attitude can put us on a winning side instead of a losing side. I recently came across this gem, which sums it up beautifully:

A loser is always part of the problem.
A winner is always part of the answer.
A loser always has an excuse.
A winner always has a program.
A loser says 'It's not my job'.
A winner says 'Let me do it for you'.
A loser sees a problem in every answer.
A winner sees an answer in every problem.
A loser sees two or three sand traps near every green.
A winner sees a green near every sand trap.
The loser says 'It may be possible but it's too difficult'.
A winner says 'It may be difficult but it's possible'.

Humour in the workplace

There's a belief that if we're serious at work we must be doing a good job. The worker who is straightfaced and always focused on the task is the one considered to be an ideal employee. The person who laughs and creates

A highly effective way to distract your thinking processes away from negative thoughts is to interrupt brain cycles with something funny or unexpected.

See if you can train yourself to inject a bit of nonsense each time you get into one of those dreary thought spirals. With practice you'll become more aware of yourself each time you start to wallow in negativity, and without conscious effort you'll be able to break in with a humorous word or association that cuts right across the way your thoughts are headed.

Once you've sidetracked yourself like this you'll have trouble getting back to worrying. I once saw a sign that read: 'If you can't convince them, confuse them!' Have fun with this idea.

humour and fun around the place is often regarded as frivolous.

To me, that's crazy logic. What is more likely to be the scenario is that the serious worker, and those around him or her, is probably stressed out. The worker who knows how to engender some light relief for themselves and others sends him- or herself and others back to work with renewed zest and a more creative attitude. A touch of humour improves performance by breaking brain patterns and stimulating approaches to the job.

When people tell me how much they enjoy their job I usually ask them if they have the opportunity for laughing and a bit of fun in the workplace, suspecting that the answer will be yes. It generally is. Conversely, where people are depressed in a job, and find it hard going, they tell me that the workplace has a dreary, serious atmosphere which discourages any light-heartedness.

The role of humour in making work more enjoyable and productive is typified by the businessman I once met on a plane. The director of the Melbourne branch of a Sydney-based company, he was a jolly man who told me (having asked what I did) that Melbourne's laughter-filled office had by far the highest sales figures nationally.

This did not surprise me. Some humour in the workplace I believe is essential to the best functioning of the individual as well as the organisation. As work takes up so much of our lives – including work at home, paid and unpaid – try introducing some measures to make your time there as pleasant as it can be.

If your place of work is already pleasant, this will add to the enjoyment. If it is not, it is especially important to introduce some humorous elements, no matter how minor. Don't wait passively, hoping a bad atmosphere will improve; find other ways to have some momentary fun. It's difficult to be the one to break the ice, but do it and be surprised that others will appreciate your gesture.

Management has an important role to play here, in letting staff know that the value of humour is understood and even promoted.

Let's not forget those who work at home, either as a householder or in a home office (the latter applies to myself when I'm not out giving talks or on the road). It's important for those who spend a lot of time in the home to also find pleasurable things to break up the day, to give ourselves some enjoyment. Breaks are essential, fun breaks send us back to the task with zest.

Putting humour to work

The following are some simple suggestions that will help you feel more positive about your work and your colleagues. You could add lots of other ways to introduce some lighter moments.

- Hang up a fun noticeboard and have everyone pin up cartoons, quips, funny sayings, jokes and cuttings that are appropriate to the organisation and to life in general. Many places start to do this or one or two people contribute from time to time, and then it tapers off. Encourage all employees to be on the lookout for new items to share and keep them updated.
- Take some photos of individuals and groups at work laughing and enjoying themselves.
- Put fun stickers on phones.
- Stick little plastic cartoon characters on your computer or other equipment.
- Bring in fun items for your desk. It doesn't matter what they are, so long as you enjoy having them around. You'll

find they are a great conversation starter. (If your work-place frowns on stickers, fun items and the like being on display, keep them in your desk drawer out of sight. Opening the drawer for a quick look from time to time will give you the same sort of boost.)

- Bring in a yo-yo or other toys that release stress. Play with them when you need a break. (I have a yo-yo that flashes and plays a tune. Kids big and small think it's great fun.)

- Plan fun activities for your lunchbreak and after work. The more negative your workplace the more important these will be.

- Encourage office humour, jokes specific to your work-place; often this can be triggered off by a secret key word.

Concern about the comfort zone also applies to people in the workplace. It is here that they particularly tell themselves they must maintain a good front, not step out of line. But reports I've read of workplaces that deliberately fostered fun in appropriate doses through joke-telling sessions, wearing funny outfits on certain days, sending funny memos or messages, social events and so on, found that the boundaries can be pushed back and nothing but good comes of it.

Give yourself a break

Much of the time work is pressured and serious, so any bit of silliness is welcomed and remembered with pleasure. Evidence shows that far from employees taking advantage of a fun-encouraging atmosphere, they are responsibly heartened by it.

Thumb wrestling is a simple, low-key, laughter-inducing activity you could introduce into your workplace or any other situation when you want a short break, to help provide a balance between the serious and the more frivolous. You will need a partner.

In this game of offence and retreat, both partners curl four fingers of one hand towards the palm, leaving the thumb sticking up. Locking both sets of fingers together, the two opposing thumbs face each other from a distance. After a quick ritual of bowing, the two thumbs 'wrestle', each trying to get on top of the other. Victory is when one person's thumb gains ascendancy and is able to rest atop the nail of the opponent's thumb.

Pinky waltzing is another such activity which also requires a partner. Curl your thumb and first three fingers inwards, extending your little finger. Your partner does the same. Then press the end of your respective little fingers together. Move your fingers and arms and bodies if you want, in a walzing motion. At the same time hum a waltz tune such as 'The Blue Danube'. The idea is to not break contact but to keep your fingers dancing as long as you are able to or want to. The point of this activity is that while you are engaged you are engrossed, and your stress levels drop.

Too shy to laugh?

Some people are shy: at work, at social events, in the classroom, virtually wherever they go. There's nothing wrong with that; it's part of what makes us all different from each other. I sympathise with those who are shy and who have to

A note for corporate people: When planning your work and your activities, and setting out your aims and your mission, what about making a kind of mission statement to do with laughter? How about incorporating one fun thing a day, a week, a month, into your working life? If you are in charge, consider extending this to your employees: having fun will generate good feelings and make colleagues more productive and contented.

grapple with the isolation it can bring. Shy children, too, often miss out on the fun things they could share with playmates.

Shy participants in my workshops have often told me that one reason they can't easily join in the fun we create is that they are afraid they will be laughed at. This fear probably goes back to painful childhood memories. Shy people are frequently sensitive souls and imagine they are the focus of attention when they are not; this can certainly inhibit their free expression of joy and laughter.

Shyness does not mean that a person is devoid of humour. Far from it. I sometimes have had great belly laughs motivated by the quiet and dry sense of humour of a 'shy' friend. The perception of shy people is just as sharp as others'; in fact it might be greater because they are often happy observing rather than having to be the centre of attention.

Shy people can also be very private people who may not feel it is safe to laugh aloud. I've noticed that being more quiet, shy people are sometimes pushed aside or talked at or over and not given a chance to catch their breath and say something.

Most of the time shyness can be lived with. If it really becomes an affliction to the point where it prohibits you from enjoying life, my advice is to seek out a counsellor or a therapist or even a trusted friend. Share with them what has led to your self-consciousness. Research shows that it is often a learned behaviour, modelled on a parent. Its cause can also lie in being 'pushed' when you were young and perhaps considered too reticent, or perhaps you were overprotected and thus never learned to trust yourself.

Whatever the reason, there is a 'you' behind this mantle who is able to relate more easily to others and to share laughs and smiles and other pleasurable, casual interactions with those around you. When you laugh you momentarily forget everything else, which is a good tactic for overcoming self-consciousness.

Too bored to laugh?

In *Laugh After Laugh* (see page 117) Raymond Moody suggests that those who feel chronically bored have a problem with their ability to enjoy themselves. I agree. Someone who knows how to have fun, to laugh, to interest and amuse themselves rarely will be bored. The complaint of boredom is really an admission that we need to add some play and humour and creativity to our lives and activities.

Our leisure time has come more and more to involve television, videos, computers and other electronic devices that tend to serve up distraction or entertainment without

Your humour is your own, unique to yourself, as personal to you as your other characteristics. Don't hold it in or censor it. You have a right to exercise your sense of humour in whatever way you like. Your perception and appreciation of the intended or unintended humour or absurdity of a situation is something you can enjoy for its own sake.

If you decide to see something as funny, it *is* funny and if that's the way you see it, no one else has the right to tell you otherwise. (Of course, it's the right of others to consider funny things that leave you cold.)

direct interaction with real people or events. As a result we are losing our capacity to look for amusement within ourselves and within the simple things around us.

I sometimes fear for those children who have grown up with video games and other high-tech items and who regard them as an essential part of life, often feeling lost if deprived of such stimulation. There's nothing wrong with this plug-in form of fun as long as both adults and children still know how to find enjoyment through their own creativity, through their sense of the ridiculous, and through shared family laughs.

Acceptable and unacceptable humour

Go ahead, let yourself burst forth with belly laughs, side-aching guffaws, giggles, titters, short barks, chuckles or lots of smiles! It's up to you. The appreciation or practice of satire, zaniness, craziness, wit, absurdity, jokes, gags and sardonic humour may all be part of the ways in which you express yourself. I encourage you to express it all, in any way you like – whatever works best for you.

But there are things that some people consider humour that I do not, and I never recommend them. Cheap laughs, especially at the expense of others, are worse than no laughs at all. The types of humour to avoid are: ridicule, cruel laughter, abuse, 'poking fun', sadistic humour, insults, humiliation, denigration, derision, 'sick' humour. These have no place in the life of a healthy individual or society. If you find yourself getting a kick out of such things you need help from someone other than myself.

5 Humour and health

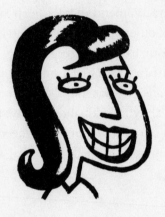

I've been very privileged over the years to be in a position to learn a lot about people and humour. One thing I've realised is the diversity of humans and their problems, and the ways they are dealt with. Another thing I've realised is the role humour can play in improving life, regardless of the individual personality or problem. The universality of humour – not of laughing at the same things, but the commonality of the capacity to find something funny – is constantly proved to me.

I quote my experiences in my groups and workshops a great deal in this book because they are a microcosm of the wider world, and what emerges there can be understood as applying to a range of broader contexts. What I have learnt has implications for applying humour in our own lives, and in particular for recognising the impact humour can have on health at all levels.

Humour for your health's sake

Taking a chance with humour for the sake of your health is always worthwhile. Below are some things participants in my workshops did which may trigger off some ideas for you. (You will see here that health at all levels is involved – physical, mental, emotional, social.)

- Jane, a shy, quiet woman who normally wouldn't have done such a thing, dared to wear a badge on Saint Patrick's Day bearing the invitation 'Kiss me, I'm Irish'. Lots of people did! Stepping out of her usual comfort zone had initially been difficult, Jane reported, but very worthwhile.

- Tony used Wiffpiff at work and his staff caught on to it and had fun with it too. He revealed that he used to get stressed out at his son borrowing his clothes and that by approaching him in fun and in Wiffpiff, he'd developed a better relationship and had been able to set the parameters he'd wanted.

- Tibor said he found the Tee hee, Ha ha exercise (see pages 18–19) valuable in stressful situations at home and at work. Fay told us she also found the exercise useful, particularly at work. Some of her workmates are now copying the idea. Ruth used Tee hee, Ha ha instead of yelling at her son, who responded a lot better to this new-style mother.

Despite his use of Tee hee, Ha ha, I had a hard time getting Tibor to loosen up so I decided to give him some pretty outrageous homework, which was fun in itself. (Homework or home play is an important aspect of the laughter classes because it's an opportunity for people to develop some humour, laughter and fun habits over a period of weeks. Most of the time each person at the end of class states their own commitment for the week. Sometimes if they are really stuck for an idea I make a relevant suggestion and ask if they are willing to try it.)

In this case I suggested to Tibor that he hug a tree during the week; he reported that he had hugged his camellia bush and the flowers had got up his nose! So I sent him back to hug a big tree and really concentrate on it. Next week he reported he had done so, but that it wasn't such a big deal for him. The great thing was that he hadn't realised just how many preconceived ideas about acceptable behaviour he'd worked through by this stage.

The final task I set him was to wear an earring in public. That took a few weeks to achieve, according to running class reports. His daughter offered to buy him an earring, his wife said she would not go out with him in public if he wore one. Tibor told us he was planning to make one. On the last night of the course, he came in sporting a tiny copper circlet in his ear. He was so proud of himself for breaking through his previous rather stodgy image that he proudly wore his jewellery out to coffee afterwards.

- Mark, who has to dress pretty conservatively for work, told us he had switched to wearing brightly coloured boxer shorts with a Mickey Mouse motif under his banker's suit.

- Debbie plucked up her courage to ask for a standing ovation (see pages 69–70) at work for something she thought deserved it. It really made a difference to her and her colleagues to do something different and affirming.
- Jennifer was a young girl who attended the course with her mother. She had recently been hospitalised after a suicide attempt and was very quiet. Jennifer reported that as a result of the workshop she now went out with friends more and was willing to take some risks in creating situations where she could have fun.
- Bonny was a school teacher who had originally booked to do a woodwork course. When that was cancelled she thought she'd give the laughter workshop a go, and participated with great joy and gusto. Bonnie found that introducing some of the ideas from the course into her own classroom was very beneficial and resulted in more cooperation and flexibility from the students. Work stress associated with teaching colleagues and stress in the home also decreased when she started to put in effect some fun and laughter-inducing activities.
- Annie had a difficult marriage and as a result had suffered poor health for many years. She threw herself into the class exercises and homework with enthusiasm, reporting that she felt in better shape mentally and physically as a result. She made a decision to live more joyfully, despite her husband.
- Mary admitted that things had got too serious for her in the last couple of years. What made her laugh most (a fact

she had now come to appreciate) was her small grand-daughter. 'I feel much happier spending the day and laughing with her than I do with anyone else. I can let myself go', she revealed.

- Sharon told us that she came along because she had read an article about laughter that said laughing stops the panic cycle. She was someone who panicked a lot and was very serious, but she noticed that when she laughed heartily she felt better about herself, and the pain in her back was less bothersome. She discovered what many others have found out: that aches and pains are worse when you pay attention to them, and an effective way to distract your-self is through laughter. Muscle tension also contributes to pain, and one of the things laughter does is decrease tension in the muscles.

- Susan reported that she was deliberately finding lots to laugh at, including minor things she had previously over-looked. 'I tripped at a meeting the other day', she said. 'I laughed, everyone else laughed, and we got off to a pro-ductive start. I also laughed recently when my budgie overbalanced and fell off its perch. The bird looked so surprised I couldn't stop laughing, even later when I recalled it.'

'Getting it fun'

Something about having fun that has become very clear from my group work and which also applies to a wider audience is the degree to which some people are constricted by their own world view. Even in simple games like 'Pass the silly face and add your own' or 'Pass on the odd sound and add your own', they need to be reminded that there is no such thing as doing it right. To the tense I say to relax, enjoy the moment and give in to the laughter our play sets off.

There is no right or wrong way of doing any of the exercises I suggest and conduct. The main thing is to do them! Life insists (in so many areas, from work to leisure to relationships) that we 'get it right', 'do it right', 'do the right thing', all of which cause a lot of stress and pressure. Laugh aerobics is about 'getting it fun', taking time out to enjoy an activity rather than having to be correct about it. There is no one to judge you.

We don't need anyone else's permission to be spontaneous and nonsensical, only our own.

Diffusing tension

For those intending to apply laugh aerobics techniques to various groups and organisations, it may help to know I never know in advance how things are going to turn out, and I am constantly amazed at how they do! Often groups one thinks would not be particularly responsive, are, while others one thinks would be, are not. Sometimes the fact that participants may already know each other or have a great deal in common (for example, from the same workplace or sharing a profession, or even an illness or condition) can work for or against the responsiveness of the group.

Attending a workshop full of strangers can be nerve-racking, especially where it is hoped you will join in something as intimate and sharing as laughter. The way I typically deal with this situation is to diffuse any discomfort or tension with humour. Light-heartedly confronting a

Kerry Cue is a well-known Australian humorous author and journalist. Last year she wrote a moving newspaper article on the death of her mother – or rather the life of her mother. The wonderful thing about this piece is the picture Kerry paints of her mother's great sense of humour and wacky approach to family life.

What Kerry had to say is so important: 'There is a message for all parents here. When you die, your children do not gather and talk about the fabulous polish on the dining-room table or the tasteful wallpaper you had in the living room. They talk about the fun. And Mum filled our lives to overflowing with laughter' (*Herald Sun*, 16 June 1995, p. 12).

Lucky for Kerry that she appreciates this, and is continuing the tradition.

situation in which people might be feeling ill-at-ease is much better than ignoring it.

For example, when Richard admitted he felt nervous and vulnerable after he discovered he was one of only two men present, I told him that their male input was all the more valuable since they were so outnumbered. Then I jokingly asked if they were single or unattached. Without waiting for a reply, I said 'Because single males at self-development courses are extremely in demand!' This bit of silliness got everyone laughing and the two men obviously became more at ease.

Positive feedback

Although I can't know what happens to participants after a course has ended, I do receive a lot of positive feedback as to how much of a difference the workshops or classes have made to people's lives. As I've experienced it, some of the things that happen during a course or workshop would seem minor to an outsider but to the person concerned they represent a significant change.

An example that comes to mind is the story of a young man who returned for a second round of classes because he enjoyed the first so much. When I initially met him he was very serious. In those early days he had been highly preoccupied with time and his watch. After a while, though, he stopped wearing his watch to the group and was able to just let time be and to savour the fun of the moment without constantly looking at his wrist.

As laughing a great deal in a group of strangers can be a rare event in life, you can be sure that people won't forget the fun they had in this way and how much better it made them feel. The experience can be a real catalyst for their taking on board some new ideas and moving their lives forward.

This adds up to a message for all of us: when you find something to laugh about, keep it in your memory in order to laugh at it again, and if it's the kind of laugh that can be shared, share it.

Humour in therapy

Although I have been trained to do so, I don't often work one-to-one with a person. For those who have deep issues to contend with, I recommend psychologists and therapists trained in these fields. My teacher in the United States, Dr Annette Goodheart, has been working for some twenty years using laughter as a carthartic process to access deeper traumas and painful experiences. She has successfully used this method with clients with cancer and AIDS, and also with victims of incest. Other therapists also work in a similar manner, although not many in this country as yet.

There is a real role for humour in therapy, which deals so much with human pain, manifesting as unhappiness, anger, depression, anxiety, repression and so on. If the therapist can introduce some lighter-hearted aspects into some sessions at an appropriate time, he or she can do a great deal for clients in showing them that it is still possible to laugh and find humour in the midst of woe, and that allowing themselves to enjoy a laugh will make them feel better. Whether the humour arises out of what the client tells the therapist or is unconnected makes no difference. The shared reaction makes for a closer relationship and improved mental health.

But humour in therapy needs to be unforced and appropriate. The therapist must be sensitive to the client, never giving the impression that he or she is being laughed at. Humour in this situation can be a very powerful tool when used with care because it can bring in a moment of lightness, giving the client a chance to stop and gain a different insight into their circumstances.

So I leave it to those who are qualified as psychotherapists and counsellors to work with clients in order to release past pain and start to reprogram some productive life skills. It's pleasing that people who have undergone or who are undergoing such therapy are coming along to my workshops as part of the recovery process. Reading this book is equally a useful thing to do in this regard.

Humour in illness

Sometimes I work with people with serious illnesses, such as cancer. Not much to laugh about there, you might think, and yet laughing can do so much good to the body and the spirit. Even though humour may be far from their minds at this time, it's very important for people who are ill to laugh.

I recall a young woman in one session who was very serious and downcast. It took a while to get her to connect with the humour that had pretty well been squashed out of her by her illness. After some of the exercises I noticed a tiny smile, then an embarrassed titter, then a genuine chuckle. By the end of our time she was laughing uproariously to the point that she couldn't speak. She came up to me afterwards and said that this was the best she had felt in a very long time.

I've worked with people from all walks of life, including nurses, who are in an occupation which certainly doesn't provide many laughs. I have found that these health professionals tend to be very stressed, and also that in workshops they find it difficult to let go and be silly and interactive because their peers are present.

One group of psychiatric nurses, I recall, really got into it, sitting on the floor like small children and finding their own way to play. At the end of the day they requested that when I return for a follow-up session I present more written information and notes about laughter and its benefits. I was happy to do so as such data would validate what they had discovered for themselves through their play activities.

The work of laughter is essentially practical. Humour needs to be actively explored, experimented with, shared and put into action. My hope is that when such professionals begin to appreciate what more fun and laughter can do in their own lives, they will work out ways to introduce it into the lives of people in institutions or clients or whenever they are in a nurturing, teaching, counselling or caring role.

The following are comments from people who took part in one of my 'Humour for Health' days.

- I am now going to be a recovering smilaholic.
- If there's a choice between laughing and crying, you may as well laugh.
- I've learnt how to make a decision to choose humour and how to overcome the fear of being silly.
- My parents made our childhood enjoyable by singing a lot. Today reminded me of that and helped me regain my sense of fun.
- I got a lot out of today. As you get older it's easier to get serious . . . That's a mistake.

Coping with grief and loss

Many of the people I encounter who are keen to add humour to their lives are coping with the process of grief and loss. Their humour has been a (hopefully temporary) casualty of this.

There's an old Chinese proverb that I like very much: 'You can't prevent the birds of sorrow from flying over your head, but you can stop them from building nests in your hair'. I have a saying of my own for times of unhappiness too: 'First do the crying, then do the laughing'.

Loss and change are part of our lives. Grief is a natural response to losing things or people that were important to us; it helps us recognise and release our feelings, and to deal with life's challenges.

Grief and loss can come in as many forms as there are people and in the way we view what happens to us and around us. However it manifests, grief is a vital sign of our humanness. The length of time it lasts and the intensity experienced varies from one person to the next. I believe we need to remember and honour that.

There comes a point, though, that whatever the loss, the grieving – at least in its acute form – needs to be done with. If it goes on too long it becomes a problem in itself. If you are grieving for a particularly lengthy time and it starts to badly affect your quality of life, I suggest you seek some grief counselling.

The grief process does come to an end, although not an abrupt one, and that is when we move on so that other people, events, situations and satisfactions can enter our lives. Just because we have lost someone or something doesn't mean that new joys, pleasures and delights don't await us.

We will attract these things when we are no longer over-shadowed by grief and sadness. Make sure you introduce

I have read studies showing that the immune systems of grieving people tend to be suppressed, and that the death rate among the bereaved during the first year of loss is more than double the normal rate. Clearly and understandably, negative thoughts, feelings and messages to oneself are at work here. Laughter and humour have their part to play at these times, helping to keep our immune systems in good shape and raising the spirits – even temporarily – when we are low.

The same need for some joyousness and fun in life applies to caregivers too, who can go downhill as rapidly as the patient if they do not nourish themselves physically, emotionally, socially – and with laughter.

more fun and laughter into your life once the utter misery of grief has abated somewhat. Your recovery will be healthier and quicker.

I can scarcely think of an occasion when humour is totally inappropriate, including those to do with grief and loss. There is a place for the appreciation of humour even when laughter itself is still at a distance. Gentle humour can lighten many situations, even sad ones. The lighter aspects of life are still there, even when we're in the midst of grief or mourning, and to pick up on them helps us along the healing process.

I found that when my mother died a couple of years ago I had a lot of tears to cry and a lot of grief to experience, but also that I was able to laugh at some of the amusing things that happened around that event. They were funny – and I let myself laugh. Perhaps some of the mirth was superficial but what mattered was that the laughter came as a relief and made the loss easier to handle.

Another good thing that came out of my attitude was that other people started telling me their stories about death and how they had handled the deaths of friends and loved ones. This openness and sharing came about because I was approachable and not wrapped up in my own sorrow.

Yet for all my emphasis on laughter, I'm also big on crying. It's just as important to cry as it is to laugh. In fact, the two are closely linked: sometimes a joyful experience can make us cry, sometimes laughter can lead to tears, and sometimes (as we have seen) when we're crying something funny can strike us and we can't help but laugh despite the tears.

So when you feel you need a crying session, don't hold yourself back. Get a box of tissues and let the tears flow freely. Know you are being human. Cry about everything you need to cry about – losses, disappointments, worries, regrets, relationships, work, children, anger, the past, parents, frustration, upsetting people, fears, health, weight, shame, pain, age, death or destruction.

Alternatively your tears may be for the plight of others, perhaps those you don't even know but whose suffering you empathise with. Or it could be that you can't even find a reason for your tears, which are, after all, a flow of feelings. They don't necessarily have to have a label for them to do you good.

After a good cry we feel calm, cleansed, relaxed – much the same as after a good laugh. In fact, if you cry hard enough, you'll feel your diaphragm going up and down like it does with helpless laughter.

We all need to cry – women *and* men; if we can let out our tears, we can also dismantle our barriers to laughter.

Laughter in recovery

One of the places in which I present workshops is an addictions clinic. I always ask 'What makes you laugh?' at the beginning of sessions to clients in recovery, as I ask it everywhere I go (it's amazing how much the responses vary). Quite often, understandably, participants reply that now that they are sober, they can't find much to laugh at. (Although one replied, 'These days, it's watching other drunks!')

It definitely can take time for people who have been through trauma or who, like addicts, have had to work through pain, anger, hurt and destructive behaviour. The recovery process is not a funny one. Yet finding – or redefining – one's humour is part of it, and not something to keep until the end. The use of humour can be a vital and integral part of recovery and letting go.

There will be some things in the lives of people who are recovering that they will not be able to change or which need to be worked on over a long period. If you can embrace these with some humour as well as let yourself be genuinely amused by what arises naturally along the road to healing and that which you seek out, you'll be doing the best for yourself. The right mental attitude, that is, a positive and cheerful one (especially when there's nothing much to be positive and cheerful about), means you are ready to take advantage of any potential humour.

I have found that the recovering addicts and others with major problems or illnesses in their lives gain a great deal from the laughter workshops, even if they aren't ready themselves to join in. To attend at all and to be comfortable witnesses to the fun and laughter of others is a positive step. As laughter is contagious, some can't help joining in despite themselves; others just find it helpful to share the atmosphere.

(I am very familiar with alcoholism and the difficulties experienced by the individuals and those close to them as my partner, a brilliant jazz musician and composer, has been grappling with the problem for many years. My association with him initially led me to my laughter work.)

Grin and bear it

Some people seem to 'grin and bear it' no matter what has happened to them and their laughing sometimes sounds out of context. Some therapists call this a 'wall of smiles' or 'hiding behind the jokes'. There is much validity in this point of view; however, I have another. I feel and recognise that this laughing stance is a coping mechanism that the individual adopts to help them deal with whatever is difficult for them. Laughing is a lot better than some of the alternatives they could turn to!

To my mind the smiling, laughing exterior is like the grown-up side taking care of the vulnerable child. For people who think they should put on a good front whatever they feel inside, it would help to be still and connect with the vulnerablility of that hurt child, and then to gently try out some playful activities.

Not so long ago I presented a laughter workshop to a group of palliative-care nurses. They are remarkable people, working with the terminally ill and dying.

Like any other group of people, they are diverse individuals and reacted to what I had to tell them in their own way. Afterwards, some told me how they deal with the stress of their occupation by being zany and silly among themselves. They have definitely found humour to be a coping tool.

I mentioned to these nurses a talk given by a rabbi I attended a couple of years ago. He said that people who had made peace within themselves and who knew that death was a transition phase left this world with a gentle 'ahhhh'. Those who had not resolved their lives and who were afraid of death left the planet, struggling, with an 'rrrrr'. One nurse told me that in her experience, people who had lived with joy and delight died easier and in peace. Those who had made life a struggle and who were full of anger hung on grimly, and death for them was difficult.

Some expert views on laughter

As we've seen, studying the benefits of laughter has become quite a business in recent years. It makes sense that the effects of humour are being studied seriously and scientifically. A lot of time and effort has gone into looking at negative states such as depression, aggression, anger and anxiety, whereas little, by contrast, has gone into the study of a healthy attribute such as laughter, which is equally a part of life. (Some of the publications to emerge from the research are very specialised, but there are a number of excellent books available, published overseas, for the general reader. You might wish to seek them out if you are interested in knowing more.)

An early publication I have found useful is *Laugh After Laugh* by Raymond A. Moody, Jr (Headwaters Press, Florida, 1978), which was one of the first books to document the value of laughter. A doctor of medicine, Moody is a great believer in the healing power of humour, and in his book he discusses patients who have 'laughed themselves back to health' or who 'have used their sense of humour as a positive and adaptive response to their illness'. Some aspects of treatment we need to leave to the medical profession, he says, but our emotions and our mental outlook are within our control, and that includes the deliberate use of humour in recovery.

He also points out the anaesthetic effect humour has on pain. I prove this each time I have to have painful injections, distracting myself with humorous thoughts and exercises such as Tee hee, Ha ha . . . They really do work.

Another writer on the subject whom I respect is Robert Holden, author of *Laughter, The Best Medicine* (Thorsons, London, 1993). Robert is a remarkable young Englishman who in 1991 helped set up the first free National Health Service laughter clinic in Birmingham, Great Britain. Two years previously he had founded the first free NHS 'stress-buster' clinic. (Incidentally, I recently learned that a humour centre has been set up in the United States to treat people who are at high risk of developing cancer.)

A study carried out recently by an Adelaide university revealed some interesting things about the role of humour among the terminally ill. It showed that laughter was useful in helping such patients deal with their illness and approaching death. Subjects in the study reported that the people around them were generally sad and wished they would lighten up! An academic connected with the study said he sees laughter as an 'emotional lifesaver' and came up with the useful idea of a 'portable humour centre' for hospitals. This would be equipped with laughter-inducing material, and could be wheeled from one bedside to another as requested.

At the British laughter clinic, staff and clients have, in Robert Holden's words, 'the opportunity to explore issues such as the pursuit of happiness, the art of joyful living, happy thinking, the inner smile, releasing the fun child, personal enjoyment and fulfilment and the therapeutic power of play, happy relationships and making fun time'.

Here in Australia we are moving towards some real recognition of the beneficial impact on health of laughter. A Laughter Factory has been opened in Adelaide, staffed by a psychologist and a comedian; it helps rehabilitate people suffering chronic pain, usually from work-related injuries. These methods, report its founders, are actually having more success in bringing about pain relief than conventional methods.

Another cheering initiative is a hospital on the south coast of Sydney which has opened a 'laughter room' for patients. Stocked with funny videos, tapes, reading matter and toys, the laughter room is also equipped with a graffiti whiteboard for writing up jokes. Hopefully other institutions in this country will follow this lead; humour rooms for patients are common in hospitals in Europe and North America. I also hope that the study of the role of humour in health will feature prominently in medical and psychotherapy courses. Until then, we need to write our own prescriptions for plenty of joyful mirth.

Allan Klein's book, *The Healing Power of Humour* (Jeremy P. Tarcher) is another useful volume to have around. It's full of hands-on ways of finding more laughter in everyday events, particularly the seemingly negative ones. In fact, its subtitle is 'Techniques for getting through loss, setbacks, upsets, disappointments, difficulties, trials, tribulations and all that not-so-funny stuff'.

In his book Klein quotes an American doctor who has studied many of the physical effects of hearty laughter and who reports that 'twenty seconds of guffawing gives the heart the same work-out as three minutes of hard rowing'.

Norman Cousins

Probably the person most connected in the public mind with the healing power of laughter is the late Norman Cousins, a respected American journalist who became ill in the 1970s with ankylosing spondylitis, a life-threatening, physically

Humour as escapism, as avoiding reality? Why not? For good reason, Jewish people have been taking refuge in it for centuries. American comic Jackie Mason (in his book *How to Talk Jewish*) explains how for Jews humour became an avenue of escape from persecution and victimisation throughout history. As a people they found that laughing at themselves, at their situation and at others, was a way of maintaining balance in the face of misery. They created a different world for themselves through humour because the one they inhabited was often so uncomfortable. As Mason puts it: 'It was a way to change the subject'. And of course, in seeking to find humour, Jewish people found it, even in unlikely circumstances.

crippling disease. Finding that his painkilling medication was actually more detrimental than the disease, and rejecting the depressing prognosis of his doctors, Mr Cousins set out to regain his health in his own way. His illness, he believed, was the outcome of too much stress, so he determined to use humour and positive emotions to try to restore the balance outside a hospital setting, which he found stressful in itself.

Norman Cousins checked himself into a hotel and, in collaboration with his sympathetic doctor who administered large doses of vitamin C, prescribed himself a positive mental attitude and massive amounts of laughter. Among other means, the latter was induced by watching lots of funny movies and amusing television shows.

A fifteen-minute session of good hearty laughter, Cousins discovered, meant he could sleep without pain for two hours; his inflammation was much reduced by the same means. Keeping up this regime, he defied medical predictions and in due course largely recovered from his illness.

Although his case was not scientifically documented, many experts who have analysed Norman Cousins' story agree that his deliberately seeking and wallowing in laughter was one of the major factors responsible for his recovery, along with a strong will to live.

Cousins' famous book, *Anatomy of an Illness*, is the culmination of his experience and his belief in the power of humour for even serious conditions. I highly recommend it.

An interesting sidelight is that in writing *Anatomy of an Illness*, Norman Cousins was not at the time making great claims for laughter as a cure-all for sickness. He wrote the book because newspaper reports at the time of his recovery had given the overwhelming impression that he had chosen laughter therapy of his own devising over conventional medical care.

In fact, Cousins' doctor was totally involved in the recovery process. In addition to the medical regime Cousins followed, he and the doctor were united in regarding laughter as standing for a whole range of positive emotions – love, hope, faith, the will to live, purpose, determination and so on – that they believed may influence good health.

It is from Norman Cousins that we have the colourful and accurate phrase 'internal jogging' to describe the effect on the body of a good laugh. (When you think about it, laughing does 'jiggle your internals', as I like to put it.)

Try it out now: laugh heartily and note how your shoulders heave, that you're breathing in a lot of air, that your innards are moving and shaking. In a corporate sense, laughter can be viewed as the managing director of the movers and shakers of our bodies.

Since that time, however, extensive research has shown that laughter can contribute to the gaining and maintenance of wellbeing. Norman Cousins didn't need to be so tentative.

Wallow in joy

A common thread through the writings discussed above is that of really feeling and expressing joy. So many of us have had the appreciation of joy and delight knocked out of us with admonishments such as: 'Don't get so excited', 'Have some decorum', 'Keep calm'. Why should we? Try a bit of raving instead, a bit of going over the top: chances are you've been behaving in such a repressed way that some healthy enthusiasm feels excessive.

When I'm in certain moods I'm pretty good (like a lot of people) at going on and on about my whinges and miseries. When I'm really bad I'm aware of actually wallowing in misery. One day when I was teaching one of my laughter classes, I began talking about the undesirability of wallowing in misery. Then I got the idea – which I shared with the group – of wallowing in joy instead (or as well as).

Why not go on and on about the good things that happen? Young children are excellent at broadcasting their pleasure: when something terrific happens or is anticipated they show their excitement, they glow, they tell everyone. When you wallow in joy, get into the feeling and the appreciation of even the smallest thing that happens to you that you like, love or feel good about. I've come to believe that it is important to connect with every bit of our joy, overlooking nothing.

If we wait for the big events to make us laugh or feel happy, the chances are we'll be waiting a long time. What do we do with ourselves in the meantime? Live in the past or fantasise about the future? Exist in the now, I tell you, and enjoy every good thing.

Joys can be public or private, major or minor. I recently experienced a private joy – not so minor – when I was on my way to conduct a laughter class. The sun was just leaving the sky, which was a beautiful hazy-pink shade. I could see the city's rooftops – all different shapes and heights and textures – and the straight lines of the TV antennas, and I began to wonder about the lives of the people living beneath them. I felt good about living in the city – a busy, crowded city green with trees and with the harbour in the distance. I felt connected to it all, and happy to be so.

Don't put it off

Don't put off the recognition of joy until you win the lottery (and the evidence shows that acquiring lots of money has very little in itself to do with joyful living) or until something desirable happens in your personal, work or social life or for anything else you hope will happen and after which you tell yourself you will feel very happy. Start today, by looking for and appreciating all that life has to offer in the present. Experience your joy wherever you find it: in nature (a sunny day, a beautiful sunset, much-needed rain), delicious food or drink, a pleasant outing, a satisfying interaction, a smile exchanged, a comfortable bed or chair, a good relationship, a happy child or pet.

The possibilities are endless. When participants in my groups have learned to stop overlooking the good things that are already there (which they often take for granted) they have come up with many more reasons for joy. Some individual reports of joy have been: buying a new piece of clothing, nails left unbitten, a leafy park, a moment of communication with a stranger, succeeding with a tricky recipe, unexpected praise or a compliment.

Being mindful of your joys helps you access the benefits of laughter. Allowing yourself to feel joyous puts you in a happier frame of mind, and when you are happy you laugh more easily and more often.

Over the years I have come to realise that to find laughter is life's on-going challenge. Life as I see it is a journey with much to be learned along the way, and laughter is our invaluable companion. As long as we remain open to our joys, there will never be a shortage of humour, fun and joy.